Pocket Guide

to

Diagnostic Tests

First Edition

William M. Detmer, MD

Assistant Clinical Professor of Medicine
University of California, San Francisco
National Library of Medicine Postdoctoral Fellow
Section on Medical Informatics, Stanford University

Stephen J. McPhee, MD

Associate Professor of Medicine
Division of General Internal Medicine
University of California, San Francisco

Diana Nicoll, MD, PhD

Clinical Professor and Vice Chair
Department of Laboratory Medicine
University of California, San Francisco
Chief, Clinical Pathology Service
Veterans Affairs Medical Center, San Francisco

Tony M. Chou, MD

Medical Chief Resident
Moffitt-Long Hospitals
University of California, San Francisco

With Associate Authors

APPLETON & LANGE
Norwalk, Connecticut

0-8385-8020-3

Copyright © 1992 by Appleton & Lange
Simon & Schuster Business and Professional Group

92 93 94 95 96 / 10 9 8 7 6 5 4 3 2 1

Prentice Hall International (UK) Limited, *London*
Prentice Hall of Australia Pty. Limited, *Sydney*
Prentice Hall Canada, Inc., *Toronto*
Prentice Hall Hispanoamericana, S.A., *Mexico*
Prentice Hall of India Private Limited, *New Delhi*
Prentice Hall of Japan, Inc., *Tokyo*
Simon & Schuster Asia Pte. Ltd., *Singapore*
Editora Prentice Hall do Brasil Ltda., *Rio de Janeiro*
Prentice Hall, *Englewood Cliffs, New Jersey*

ISBN: 0-8385-8020-3
ISSN: 1061-3463

Table of Contents

Associate Authors

Susan D. Wall, MD
Associate Professor of Radiology
University of California, San Francisco
Assistant Chief, Radiology Service
Veterans Affairs Medical Center, San Francisco

Cheryl L. Futerman, MD
Clinical Instructor in Radiology
University of California, San Francisco
Veterans Affairs Medical Center, San Francisco

Preface

Purpose

This book is intended to serve as a pocket reference manual for medical and other health professional students, house officers, and practicing physicians. It is a quick reference guide to the selection and interpretation of commonly used diagnostic tests, including bedside diagnostic tests, laboratory tests (chemistry, hematology, and immunology), microbiology tests (bacteriology, virology, and serology), and diagnostic imaging tests (plain radiography, CT, MRI, and ultrasonography). Though the *Guide* focuses almost exclusively on diagnosis, treatment alternatives are presented in a few sections (eg, in the microbiology chapter) where diagnosis and treatment are closely related.

This book will enable readers to understand commonly used diagnostic tests and diagnostic approaches to common disease states. It recognizes the provider's need to understand these tests and approaches so that rational therapeutic approaches can be developed.

Outstanding Features

- Over 300 tests are presented in a concise, consistent, and readable format.
- Fields covered include internal medicine, pediatrics, general surgery, neurology, and gynecology.
- Costs and risks of various procedures and tests are emphasized.
- Literature references are included for most diagnostic tests.
- An index for quick reference is included inside the back cover.

Organization

This pocket reference manual is not intended to include all diagnostic tests or disease states. Rather, the authors have selected those tests and diseases that are most common and relevant to the general practice of medicine.

The *Guide* is divided into 11 sections:

1. Basic Principles of Diagnostic Test Use and Interpretation
2. Performance of Common Bedside Diagnostic Procedures
3. Common Laboratory Tests: Selection and Interpretation
4. Therapeutic Drug Monitoring: Principles and Test Interpretation
5. Microbiology: Test Selection and Treatment
6. Diagnostic Imaging: Test Selection and Interpretation
7. Diagnostic Tests in Differential Diagnosis
8. Diagnostic Algorithms
9. Nomograms and Reference Material
10. Organization of Laboratory Data: Pocket Patient Cards

Intended Audience

In this era of rapidly changing medical technology, many new diagnostic tests are being introduced every year and are replacing older tests as they are shown to be more sensitive, specific, or cost-effective. In this environment, students, house officers, and practicing physicians are looking for a pocket reference on diagnostic tests.

Medical students will find the concise summary of diagnostic laboratory, microbiologic, and imaging studies in this pocket-sized book of great help during clinical ward rotations. The Patient Pocket Cards will enable them to easily organize and carry with them their patients' clinical data.

Busy house officers will find the clear organization and citations to the current literature useful in devising proper patient management.

Practitioners (internists, family physicians, pediatricians, surgeons, and other specialists who provide generalist care) may use the *Guide* as a refresher manual to update their understanding of laboratory tests and diagnostic approaches.

Nurses and other health practitioners will find the format and scope of the *Guide* valuable for understanding the use of laboratory tests in patient management.

Acknowledgments

We wish to thank our associate authors, Susan D. Wall, MD, and Cheryl L. Futerman, MD, for their contributions to this book. In addition, we are grateful to the many physician and student reviewers who contributed useful suggestions. In particular, we would like to thank Ralph Cavalieri, MD, Mark Chesnutt, MD, Laurence Corash, MD, Kenneth Feingold, MD, Peter Fitzgerald, MD, PhD, Stephen Gerard, MD, PhD, James Grendell, MD, Keith Hadley, MD, Jaisri Lingappa, MD, Theodore Kurtz, MD, Scott Monroe, MD, Steven Porter, MD, Lynn Pulliam, PhD, Jay Sanford, MD, Merle Sande, MD, Daniel Stites, MD, Gordon Strewler, MD, Lawrence Tierney, MD, Pearl Toy, MD, James Tulsky, MD, Michael Winter, PharmD, and Theresa Wright, MD. The authors would also like to thank Suzie Ushijima and Shelley Stork, who helped prepare the manuscript.

We welcome comments and recommendations from our readers for future editions.

William M. Detmer, MD
Stephen J. McPhee, MD
Diana Nicoll, MD, PhD
Tony M. Chou, MD

San Francisco
April, 1992

1 Basic Principles of Diagnostic Test Use and Interpretation

USES OF DIAGNOSTIC TESTS

Diagnostic tests are generally used for three purposes.

Screening tests are used for identifying risk factors for a given disease in asymptomatic persons, or for detecting occult disease. Early identification of risk factors may allow intervention that could prevent disease occurrence; early detection of occult disease may reduce disease morbidity and mortality.

Diagnostic tests are used to help establish or exclude the presence of disease in symptomatic persons. Such tests may assist in diagnosis, in differential diagnosis, or in determining disease stage or activity.

Management tests are used to evaluate disease severity and prognosis, to monitor the course of disease (ie, progression, stability, or resolution), or to help select and adjust therapy.

ATTRIBUTES OF DIAGNOSTIC TESTS

Test precision is a measure of a test's reproducibility when it is repeated on the same sample. An imprecise test is one that yields widely varying results on repeated measurements.

Test accuracy reflects the ability of the test to identify the true value. An inaccurate test is one that consistently differs from the true value, even though the results may be reproducible.

Reference ranges are determined for each test by the laboratory; test results can be interpreted only by comparison with laboratory-specific reference ranges. Laboratories usually define reference ranges by testing healthy volunteers, plotting a frequency distribution of the results, and calculating the mean and standard deviation. The results of a quantitative laboratory test sometimes conform roughly to a gaussian bell-shaped distribution (Figure 1–1). Reference ranges may be reported as those values within 2 standard deviations of the mean (or the range of values within which 95% of healthy individuals fall).

The distribution of laboratory test values for healthy individuals usually overlaps that for diseased persons, so that establishment of the upper limit of normal will affect the sensitivity and specificity of the test (Figure 1–2).

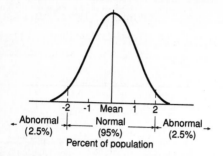

Figure 1–1. The normal range is often defined as values within 2 standard deviations of the mean (shown as –2 and 2) in a population of healthy volunteers.

Test sensitivity is the probability that a test result will be *positive* if the disease being investigated is *present* (Figure 1–3). A test with positive (abnormal) results in all patients with a given disease would have perfect (100%) sensitivity (ie, no false-negative results). A perfectly sensitive test can exclude ("rule out") a possible diagnosis if the result is negative (normal).

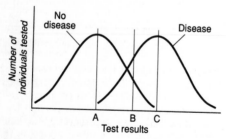

Figure 1–2. Hypothetical distribution of test results for healthy and diseased individuals. The position of the "cutoff point" between "normal" and "abnormal" (or "negative" and "positive") test results determines the test's sensitivity and specificity. If point **A** is the cutoff point, the test would have 100% sensitivity but low specificity. If point **C** is the cutoff point, the test would have 100% specificity but low sensitivity. For most tests, the cutoff point is usually somewhere in between points **A** and **C**, at a point **B**. The importance of maximizing either sensitivity or specificity depends on why the test is usually ordered and the relative importance of false-positive and false-negative results. (Modified and reproduced, with permission, from Griner PF et al: Selection and interpretation of diagnostic tests and procedures: Principles and applications. Ann Intern Med 1981;84[4 Part 2]:453.)

Disease

	Present	Absent
Positive (abnormal)	a	b
Negative (normal)	c	d

Test result

Definitions

$$\text{Sensitivity} = \frac{a}{a+c} \times 100\%$$

$$= \frac{\text{Number of persons with disease with positive tests}}{\text{Total number of persons with disease}}$$

$$\text{Specificity} = \frac{d}{b+d} \times 100\%$$

$$= \frac{\text{Number of persons without disease with negative tests}}{\text{Total number of persons without disease}}$$

$$\text{Positive predictive value} = \frac{a}{a+b} \times 100\%$$
$$= \text{Probability of disease if test positive}$$

$$\text{Negative predictive value} = \frac{d}{c+d} \times 100\%$$
$$= \text{Probability of no disease if test negative}$$

Figure 1–3. Potential relationships between disease and test results.

Test specificity is the probability that a test result will be *negative* if the disease being investigated is *not present* (Figure 1–3). A test with negative (normal) results in all patients without a given disease would have perfect (100%) specificity (ie, no false-positive results). A perfectly specific test can confirm ("rule in") a possible diagnosis if the result is positive (abnormal).

Predictive values of a test are expressed either as positive or negative. The *positive predictive value* of a test is the probability that the patient has the disease if the test result is positive; the *negative predictive value* of a test is the probability that the patient is free of the disease if the test result is negative (Figure 1–3).

Bayes' theorem states that the predictive values (positive and negative) of a test relate not only to the characteristics of the test but also to the frequency of the disease in the population being tested (**disease prevalence**). This means that physicians must take into account not only the sensitivity and specificity of the test ordered but also the known or estimated probability that the disease is present.

Table 1–1. Effect of Prior Probability (Prevalence) on Predictive Value of Positive Test Results.

Prior Probability (Prevalence), %	Predictive Value of a Positive Test When Sensitivity = 95% and Specificity = 95%
0.1	1.9
1	16.1
2	27.9
5	50.0
50	95.0

Pretest probability (likelihood) of disease is the clinician's estimate of whether a disease is present based on data from the history and physical examination.

When the pretest likelihood is high, a positive (abnormal) test result helps to confirm the diagnosis but a negative (normal) result does not rule out the diagnosis. When the pretest likelihood is low, a negative (normal) result helps to exclude the diagnosis but a positive (abnormal) result is not particularly helpful. Tests are most likely to be useful when the diagnosis is truly uncertain (pretest likelihood about 50%). Laboratory tests add little when the diagnosis is either extremely unlikely or almost certain. Table 1–1 shows the effects of various prior probabilities (prevalences) on the predictive value of positive tests for a diagnostic test with a sensitivity and specificity of 95%. Note that if the prior probability of disease is low (eg, < 5%), a positive test is more likely to be a false-positive than a true-positive.

Summary

Diagnostic tests, when used appropriately, can assist in diagnosis, establish prognosis, guide therapy, lead to a better understanding of the disease process, and benefit the patient. However, if ordered without clinical indication, diagnostic tests are likely to lead to confusion.

References

Griner PF et al: Selection and interpretation of diagnostic tests and procedures: Principles and applications. Ann Intern Med 1981;84(4, Part 2):453.

Johns RJ, Fortuin NJ, Wheeler PS: The collection and evaluation of clinical information. In: *The Principles and Practice of Medicine*, 22nd ed. Appleton & Lange, 1988.

Sox HC et al: Sensitivities and specificities of diagnostic tests. In: *Medical Decision Making*. Butterworths, 1988.

2 Performance of Common Bedside Diagnostic Procedures[1]

This chapter contains information on how to perform common bedside diagnostic procedures. Though the focus is mostly on the performance of procedures, some sections include information on interpretation.

---

[1] Chapter modified, with permission, from Ho MT, Saunders CE (editors): *Current Emergency Diagnosis and Treatment*, 3rd ed. Appleton & Lange, 1990; and Krupp MA et al: *Physician's Handbook*, 21st ed. Lange, 1985.

1. SAFETY CONSIDERATIONS

General Safety Considerations

All patient specimens are potentially infectious; therefore the following precautions should be taken:

Universal body fluid and needle stick precautions must be observed at all times.

Disposable gloves, gown, mask, and goggles should be worn when collecting specimens.

Gloves should be changed and hands washed after contact with each patient. Dispose of gloves in an appropriate biohazard waste container.

Any spills should be cleaned up with 10% bleach solution.

Handling and Disposing of Needles

Do not resheath needles.

Discard needles only into designated containers.

Do not remove a used needle from a syringe by hand. The needle may be removed using a specially designed waste collection system or the entire assembly may (if disposable) be discarded as a unit into a designated container.

When obtaining blood cultures, it is hazardous and unnecessary to change needles.

Do not put phlebotomy or other equipment on the patient's bed.

Informed Consent

Remember that every diagnostic procedure carries risks of possible complications.

Explain the planned procedure to the patient to facilitate cooperation and to help alleviate anxiety.

Most hospitals require written permission documenting informed consent of the patient for major invasive procedures, such as thoracentesis, paracentesis, and lumbar puncture.

Identification of Specimens

Positively identify the patient before obtaining the specimen (if the patient is not known to you, ask the name and check the wristband).

Label each specimen container with the patient's name and identification number.

Specimen Tubes

Standard specimen tubes are now widely available and are easily identified by the color of the stopper (see also p 39):

Red top tubes contain no anticoagulants or preservatives and are used for chemistry tests.

Marbled top tubes contain material that allows ready separation of serum and clot by centrifugation.

Lavender top tubes contain EDTA and are used for hematology tests (eg, blood or cell counts, differentials).

Green top tubes contain heparin and are used for tests that require plasma or anticoagulation.

Blue top tubes contain citrate and are used for coagulation tests.

Gray top tubes contain fluoride and are used for some chemistry tests (eg, glucose) if the specimen cannot be analyzed immediately.

When collecting multiple specimens, fill sterile tubes used for bacteriologic tests, then tubes without additives (ie, red top tubes) before filling those with additives to avoid the potential for bacterial contamination or transfer of anticoagulants, etc. However, be certain to fill tubes containing anticoagulants before the blood specimen clots.

The recommended order of filling tubes is (by type and color): (1) blood culture, (2) red top, (3) blue top, (4) green top, (5) purple top.

2. UPPER EXTREMITY VENIPUNCTURE

Indications

To obtain venous blood for laboratory analysis.

Contraindications

Cellulitis, phlebitis, venous obstruction, lymphangitis, or arteriovenous fistula or shunt at proposed venipuncture site.

Intravenous catheter distal to proposed site. To avoid spurious test results from IV solutions, do not draw blood above an intravenous catheter or infusion site.

Approach to the Patient

Label each tube with the patient's name and identification number (see p 6).

Put on gloves, gown, and goggles.

Place the patient in a comfortable sitting or lying (never standing) position, with the upper extremity extended and firmly supported (eg, by a pillow or bedside table).

Apply a tourniquet above the antecubital fossa tight enough to occlude venous return, but not enough to cause discomfort or arterial obstruction. Do not leave a tourniquet on for more than 2 minutes.

Have the patient open and close the fist to pump blood from muscles into veins.

Locate an appropriate vein, such as the superficial basilic or cephalic vein (Figure 2–1A).

Procedural Technique

Palpate the antecubital fossa with the tip of your index finger, feeling for the buoyant resilience of a distended vein.

Cleanse the skin with iodine or alcohol. (Use iodine if blood is being obtained for culture, alcohol if serum is being obtained.)

Grasp the syringe (or Vacutainer) in your dominant hand while using the index finger of your other hand to palpate the vein and put traction on the vein by pulling it toward yourself. However, do not touch the venipuncture site after cleansing it.

Align the needle along the course of the vein, with the bevel facing up. Push the needle quickly and smoothly through the skin at a 10–20 degree angle and advance it into the vein lumen (Figure 2–1B).

Pull the syringe plunger out away from the needle (or push the Vacutainer tube onto the needle) and observe for blood flow into the syringe (or tube).

Withdraw the amount of blood required with a steady, even pull on the plunger. (When too much force is applied, the vein will collapse. If this occurs, stop to allow the vein to fill, then resume pulling with less force.)

When enough blood has been obtained, remove the tourniquet, and then withdraw the needle quickly and smoothly.

Ask the patient to apply immediate firm pressure on a 2 × 2 gauze

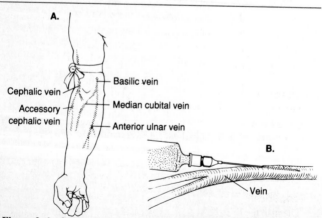

Figure 2–1. A: Principal veins of the arm (highly variable). **B:** Needle placement in a vein. (Reproduced, with permission, from: Krupp MA et al: *Physician's Handbook*, 21st ed. Lange, 1985.)

placed directly over the insertion site for 3–5 minutes. Inspect the puncture site. If bleeding has stopped, apply an adhesive bandage.

Use a new needle if a second venipuncture is required.

Possible Complications

Hematoma at or bleeding from puncture site.

Thrombophlebitis.

Infection (septic phlebitis).

Vasovagal syncope.

Specimen Handling

Fill the blood tubes completely and tilt each tube containing anticoagulant or preservative to mix thoroughly. Place any specimens on ice as required.

Do not remove the needle from the syringe. Properly dispose of the needle, then gloves (see p 6).

3. RADIAL ARTERY PUNCTURE

Indications

To obtain arterial blood for blood gas analysis and pH determination.

To obtain blood for laboratory analysis when phlebotomy sites are unavailable.

Contraindications

Absence of palpable radial artery pulse, or positive Allen test (indicating that only one artery supplies hand).

Cellulitis over proposed radial artery puncture site.

Arteriovenous fistula or shunt.

Severe thrombocytopenia (platelet count < 20,000/μL) or prothrombin time or partial thromboplastin time prolongation > 1.5 times control (relative contraindication).

Approach to the Patient

Put on gloves, gown and goggles.

Have the patient sit with the upper extremity extended, volar side up, on a stable surface (eg, bedside table or side of bed).

Locate the radial artery maximum pulsation just proximal to the wrist (Figure 2–2). The radial artery runs between the styloid process of the radius and the flexor carpi radialis tendon.

Procedural Technique

Cleanse the skin with iodine or alcohol.

Palpate the radial artery under the ball of your nondominant index finger, by slowly moving the finger from side to side. Place your index and middle fingers over the point of maximum pulsation (Figure 2–2).

Holding the heparinized syringe and needle perpendicularly to the arm, insert the needle into the skin and guide it toward the point of maximum arterial pulsation (Figure 2–2). Push the needle smoothly through the arterial wall and observe for a sudden gush of blood into the syringe.

The force of arterial pulsation should fill the syringe, but if necessary gently pull the plunger out away from the needle.

When enough blood (for blood gases, usually 1–2 mL) has been obtained, withdraw the needle quickly and smoothly, and apply immediate firm pressure on a 2 × 2 gauze placed directly over the insertion site for 10 minutes.

Return in 15 minutes to check the patient's hand for adequate perfusion and the wrist for a hematoma.

Possible Complications

Hematoma at or bleeding from puncture site.

Thrombosis of radial artery.

Infection.

Specimen Handling

Evacuate air bubbles by holding the syringe upright and tapping gently on its side to allow bubbles to collect near the needle hub, then pushing gently on the plunger.

Remove the needle carefully and dispose of it properly (see p 6).

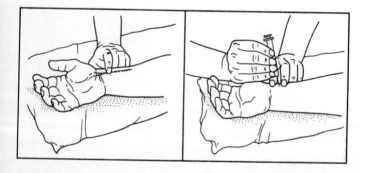

Figure 2–2. Technique of radial artery puncture. The nondominant index and middle fingers are positioned over the artery at the point of maximal pulsation. (Reproduced, with permission, from: Ho MT et al: *Current Emergency Diagnosis & Treatment*, 3rd ed. Appleton & Lange, 1990.)

Place the rubber cap over the hub, label the specimen with the patient's name and identification number, and place the sample on ice for immediate delivery to the laboratory.

Arterial blood should be sent for pH, PO_2, and PCO_2. (See Acid-base nomogram, p 261, for guide to interpretation.)

4. THORACENTESIS

Indications

To obtain pleural fluid for diagnostic tests.

To relieve respiratory distress by evacuating fluid in pleural space.

Contraindications

Severe thrombocytopenia (platelet count < 20,000/µL) or prothrombin time or partial thromboplastin time prolongation > 1.5 times control (correct these abnormalities first, if possible).

Agitated, uncooperative patient (relative contraindication).

Approach to the Patient

Label each specimen tube with the patient's name and identification number (see p 6).

Thoracentesis is usually performed by a posterior approach. The patient should be seated on the edge of the bed or gurney with arms and trunk bent forward over a bedside stand, supported by the elbows or pillows. (If unable to sit, the patient should lie at the edge of the bed on the affected side with the ipsilateral arm over the head and the midaxillary line accessible for insertion of the needle. Elevating the head of the bed to 30 degrees sometimes helps.)

Locate the pleural effusion and estimate the level of the fluid meniscus by careful percussion of both sides or by ultrasonography. Mark the top of the dullness (eg, by scratching or indenting the skin). Access to the pleural space is gained through the intercostal space (Figure 2–3). The needle is inserted over the top of the rib to avoid the intercostal nerves and blood vessels that run on its underside. Remember that the dome of the diaphragm is highest posteriorly, occasionally as high as the seventh intercostal space.

Procedural Technique

Observe sterile technique (don cap, mask, gloves, and gown).

Arrange equipment on a sterile field on a bedside stand.

Select the thoracentesis site below the level of the fluid meniscus in the midposterior line (posterior insertion) or midaxillary line (lateral insertion).

Sterilize the skin around the insertion site with iodine.

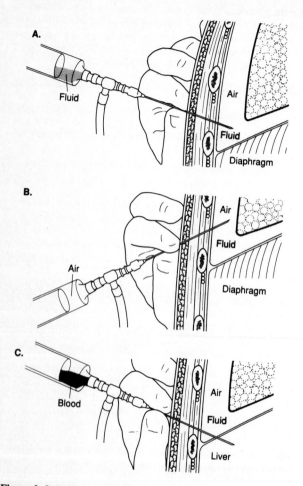

Figure 2–3. Technique of thoracentesis, using a regular needle (not catheter-clad). **A:** Successful tap, with fluid obtained. Note the position of the needle in relation to the intercostal nerve and blood vessels. **B:** Air is obtained if the needle position is too high (lung is punctured or preexisting pneumothorax, as pictured). **C:** Bloody fluid is obtained if the needle position is too low (liver or spleen is punctured). (Reproduced, with permission, from: Chesnutt MS, Dewar TD [editors]: *Office and Bedside Procedures.* Appleton & Lange, 1992.)

Drape the patient.

Anesthetize the skin over the insertion site with 1% lidocaine using a 5-mL syringe and a 25- or 27-gauge needle; then anesthetize the superior surface of the rib and the parietal pleura.

Catheter-Clad Needle (eg, Angiocath) Insertion

Attach a 30-mL standard syringe to the catheter-clad needle (usually 16- to 18-gauge Angiocath).

While exerting steady pressure on the patient's back with the non-dominant hand, insert the needle through the skin over the rib selected. Advance the needle until it encounters the superior aspect of the rib.

Have the patient take a deep breath and hold it against a closed glottis.

Advance the needle over the top of the rib and through the pleura, maintaining constant, gentle suction on the syringe.

When pleural fluid gushes into the syringe, advance the needle slightly, then angle it downward, and advance the catheter over the needle downward into the base of the pleural space.

Keeping the syringe connected, have the patient exhale and breathe normally.

Have the patient take a deep breath again and hold it; disconnect the syringe, withdraw the needle, and insert a 3-way stopcock into the catheter hub. Make sure the stopcock valve is set to occlude the catheter port. Then have the patient resume normal breathing.

Connect a 30-mL Luer-Lok syringe to one port of the 3-way stop-cock and (if needed) intravenous tubing to the other.

Turn the stopcock valve to connect the syringe with the catheter and withdraw fluid from the pleural space. Set the valve to occlude the catheter port, disconnect the syringe, and inject pleural fluid into specimen tubes for diagnostic tests (see below).

Reconnect the syringe, open the stopcock to the syringe, and with-draw more fluid. Then turn the stopcock to connect the syringe to the tubing and empty the syringe through the tubing into an empty cytology bottle.

Repeat this procedure to withdraw as much fluid as possible (but generally not more than 1 L with each thoracentesis). To com-pletely evacuate the pleural space, you may need to rock the patient gently from side to side.

When no more fluid can be withdrawn, have the patient take a deep breath and hold it, then quickly withdraw the catheter. Cover the insertion site with a sterile occlusive dressing.

Obtain an upright portable (expiratory) chest x-ray to check for pos-sible pneumothorax and residual fluid.

Needle-Clad Catheter (eg, Intracath) Insertion

The procedure is the same as described above, except:

After inserting the needle (usually from a 14- to 16-gauge Intracath) into the pleural space and withdrawing fluid, attach a Kelley clamp to the needle to prevent it from being inserted too far.

Have the patient take a deep breath and hold it, then quickly disconnect the syringe, and insert the catheter through the needle, aiming downward toward the base of the pleural space. Withdraw the needle, leaving the catheter inside the pleural space. Occlude the lumen of the catheter with a closed stopcock, and have the patient resume normal breathing.

Follow the remaining steps as above.

Possible Complications

Pneumothorax, including tension pneumothorax.

Hemothorax, bleeding.

Infection (empyema).

Laceration of intraabdominal viscera (eg, liver, spleen).

Specimen Handling

Fill the tubes with the required amount of pleural fluid and tilt each tube containing anticoagulant or preservative to mix thoroughly. Dispose of the needle, then gloves properly (see p 6).

Check that each tube is properly labeled.

Pleural fluid should be sent to the laboratory for: cell count and differential (in purple top tube); protein and glucose (red top); culture and Gram's stain (sterile tube); and, if neoplasm is suspected, for cytology (generally requires 1 L of fluid in cytology bottle). (For guide to interpretation, see Pleural fluid profiles, p 232.)

5. ABDOMINAL PARACENTESIS

Indications

To obtain ascitic fluid for laboratory analysis (eg, in diagnosis of etiology of new ascites, in suspected bacterial peritonitis, or in suspected intraabdominal hemorrhage from trauma).

To lower intraabdominal pressure (eg, in relief of symptoms in patients with tense ascites).

Contraindications

Marked bowel distention (correct distension first, using NG suction or rectal tube decompression).

Previous abdominal surgery (scar near proposed insertion site).

Severe thrombocytopenia (platelet count < 20,000/μL) or prothrom-

bin time or partial thromboplastin time prolongation > 1.5 times
control (relative contraindication; correct these abnormalities first,
if possible).

Approach to the Patient

Label each tube with the patient's name and identification number
(see p 6).

Be sure the patient's bladder is empty.

Place the patient supine at the edge of the bed (right side of bed if
you are right-handed), with the trunk elevated 45 degrees.

Access to the peritoneal space is usually obtained through the midline linea alba about halfway between the symphysis pubis and
umbilicus, or through the fascia bordering the rectus sheath in the
left lower quadrant (Figure 2–4). Tip the patient 30 degrees to that
side if performing paracentesis of a lower quadrant.

Procedural Technique

Observe sterile technique (don mask, gloves, gown, and goggles).

Arrange equipment on a sterile field on a bedside stand.

Select the paracentesis site in the midline or lower quadrant.

Sterilize the skin around the insertion site with iodine.

Drape the patient.

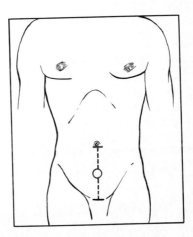

Figure 2–4. Insertion site for abdominal paracentesis. (Reproduced,
with permission, from: Dunphy JE et al: *Current Surgical Diagnosis &
Treatment,* 5th ed. Lange, 1981.)

Anesthetize the skin over the insertion site with 1% lidocaine using a 5-mL syringe and a 25- or 27-gauge needle. Change to a 22-gauge needle, then anesthetize down to and including the peritoneum.

Attach a 19- or 20-gauge catheter-clad needle (eg, Angiocath) to a 50-mL syringe. (In patients with severe coagulation disorders, use a 22-gauge needle. In markedly obese patients, a 3-1/2 inch 20- or 22-gauge spinal needle may be needed.)

Puncture the anesthetized skin. Keeping the needle perpendicular to the abdominal wall, advance the needle slowly until fluid flows freely into the syringe. While advancing the syringe, maintain constant, gentle suction. In tense ascites, try to Z-track the needle to minimize persistent leakage of ascites. (To Z-track, after puncturing the skin but before puncturing the subcutaneous tissue, move the needle and syringe 0.5–1 cm laterally while maintaining the perpendicular approach.)

For diagnostic paracentesis, collect 50 mL of ascitic fluid.

For relief of ascites, remove up to 1 L of fluid.

When enough fluid has been withdrawn, quickly withdraw the catheter. Cover the insertion site with a sterile pressure dressing. If leaking of ascitic fluid occurs, close the paracentesis track with a mattress stitch.

Possible Complications

Perforation or laceration of abdominal or pelvic viscera (eg, gut or bladder).

Bleeding.

Infection (peritonitis).

Specimen Handling

Fill the tubes completely with pleural fluid and tilt each tube containing anticoagulant or preservative to mix thoroughly. Properly dispose of the needle, then gloves (see p 6).

Check that each tube is properly labeled.

Ascitic fluid should be sent to the laboratory for: cell count and differential (purple top tube); protein and amylase (red top); Gram's stain and culture (sterile tube); and, if neoplasm is suspected, cytology (requires up to 1 L in cytology bottle). (See Ascitic fluid profiles, p 224, for guide to interpretation.)

6. INSERTION OF (FOLEY) BLADDER CATHETER

Indications

To drain the urinary bladder (diagnostic or therapeutic drainage).

To enable frequent, reliable assessment of urinary output (eg, shock).

Contraindications (Relative)

Recent urethral surgery.

Suspected or known urethral trauma (bloody discharge from the urethral meatus or a free-floating prostate on rectal examination).

Inability to pass a catheter easily.

Approach to the Patient

A Foley catheter consists of a double-lumen rubber tube with an inflatable rubber balloon near its tip. The larger lumen is for bladder drainage, the smaller is for inflation of the retaining balloon. (Some indwelling catheters have a third lumen for constant bladder irrigation.) Foley catheters are of standard length (46 cm) but different diameters (numerically graded by the French system) and balloon sizes (5 mL and 30 mL). A 14F or 18F catheter with a 5-mL balloon is generally used for routine, short-term catheterization. Men with prostatic hypertrophy may require larger catheters (eg, 20F or 22F).

Females: The female urethra is short, exits the bladder at the trigone, and terminates at the meatus. The meatus is located at the superior fornix of the vulva, above the vaginal opening and below the clitoris. For catheter insertion, the patient should be in the lithotomy position (or with the soles of the feet pressed together).

Males: The male urethra is long, exits the bladder at the trigone, passes through the prostate, and runs the length of the penis to terminate at the meatus. For catheter insertion, the patient should be supine, with the penis held upright (perpendicular to the abdomen) (Figure 2–5).

Procedural Technique

Place the open catheter tray and selected catheter on a sterile field on the bedside stand. Squeeze lubricant onto the sterile field.

Put on gloves and gown.

Drape the perineal area.

Fill a syringe with 5 mL of sterile water for inflating the balloon.

Open the antiseptic packet, soak the cotton swabs with the antiseptic.

Females: Stand on the patient's right side, spread the labia with your left hand, and identify the urethral meatus. Cleanse the area with the cotton swabs, using front to back strokes. Keep the labia spread apart with your left hand.

Males: Stand on the patient's right side, grasp the penis with your left hand, holding it upright, perpendicular to the abdomen. Cleanse the glans and urethral meatus with 3 or 4 swabs.

Grasp the Foley catheter with your right hand, making a loop for easier handling, and coat the tip with lubricant.

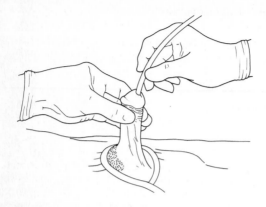

Figure 2–5. Technique of bladder (Foley) catheter placement.
(Reproduced, with permission, from: Chesnutt MS, Dewar TD [editors]:
Office and Bedside Procedures. Appleton & Lange, 1992.)

Insert the catheter tip into the urethral meatus, advance it until urine
returns, then advance it another 4–5 cm into the bladder (females)
or, using successive, steady motions, to the hilt (males) to ensure
that the balloon is not inflated in the urethra.

Inflate the balloon with the sterile water, then withdraw the catheter
gently to pull the balloon snugly against the trigone.

Collect a urine specimen in a sterile container; then connect the catheter to a urinary drainage bag. Tape the Foley catheter and drainage tube to the upper thigh, leaving enough slack to allow easy
abduction of the leg.

Possible Complications

Urethral or bladder injury.

Bleeding.

Infection (urinary tract infection).

Specimen Handling

Urine should be sent to the laboratory for: routine urinalysis, including both dipstick examination (see Table 2–1, p 34) and microscopic examination for cells, casts, crystals, and bacteria (see
Figure 2–14, p 33); culture and Gram's stain; and, if neoplasm is
suspected, for cytology. (See also p 31 for technique of urinalysis,
and p 244 for guide to interpretation of urine composition in various disease states.)

7. LUMBAR PUNCTURE (LP)

Indications

To obtain cerebrospinal fluid (CSF) for laboratory analysis.

To administer antimicrobial or chemotherapeutic agents.

To lower CSF pressure (in benign intracranial hypertension or pseudotumor cerebri).

Contraindications

Soft tissue infections of the lumbar area (perform cervical or cisternal puncture instead).

Suspected intracranial mass lesion, eg, papilledema or focal cerebral defects(perform a CT or MRI scan of head before attempting LP).

Suspected spinal cord mass lesion (perform myelography instead).

Severe thrombocytopenia (platelet count < 20,000/μL) or prothrombin time or partial thromboplastin time prolongation > 1.5 times control (relative contraindications; correct these abnormalities first, if possible).

Approach to the Patient

Label each tube with the patient's name and identification number (see p 6).

Have the patient lie in lateral decubitus position, facing away from you. Put the patient in a fetal position (forehead bent toward knees and knees drawn up to abdomen) with the lumbar area at the edge of the right side of the bed. Put the patient's head on a pillow to keep the craniospinal axis parallel to the bed. The line of the patient's shoulders and pelvis must be perpendicular to the bed. Keep the patient's knees and ankles aligned to prevent pelvic rotation. Have an assistant stand by to help the patient maintain the proper position (Figure 2–6) and to assist with capping tubes.

(Less commonly, LP is performed with the patient sitting. Have the patient sit facing away from you, bent over a bedside table.)

Raise the bed until the patient's lumbar area is at your mid-chest level when you are seated and ready to perform the LP.

The L3–L4 interspace, the most common insertion site for lumbar puncture, is at the level of the iliac crests (Figure 2–6). (The L4–L5 interspace may also be used.) The needle should enter the subarachnoid space below the level of the conus medullaris, which extends to L1–L2 in most adults and to L2–L3 in children. With the patient properly positioned, find the posterior iliac crests, and palpate the spine at this level to locate the L3–L4 interspace. Find the exact midpoint of the interspace between the spinous processes. Mark the insertion site by scratching or indenting the skin.

Procedural Technique

Observe sterile technique (don mask, gloves, gown, and goggles).

Arrange equipment on a sterile field on a bedside stand. Assemble the manometer and stopcock so that the channel from the spinal needle to the manometer is open, and open the specimen tubes.

Sterilize the skin around the insertion site with iodine.

Place a sterile drape under the patient, extending over the edge of the bed, and tape a second drape over the top of the sterilized site.

Anesthetize the skin over the insertion site with 1% lidocaine using a 5-mL syringe and a 25- or 27-gauge needle. Change to a 22-gauge needle, then anesthetize between the spinous processes.

Hold the 20- or 22-gauge spinal needle between the index and middle fingers, with your thumb over the stylet (or hold it in both hands, if necessary). Avoid touching the tip or shaft of the needle.

With the bevel of the needle facing up, puncture the anesthetized skin at the midline insertion site. Keeping the needle perpendicular to a line connecting the iliac crests, advance it slowly, aiming toward the umbilicus (in adults, aim about 30 degrees rostrally; in infants, aim nearer to the perpendicular; in the elderly, aim about 45 degrees rostrally). Keep the patient's back perpendicular to the bed and the long axis of the needle parallel to the bed.

Advance the needle and stylet slowly, frequently checking the position of the needle (by withdrawing the stylet). There is often a "pop" as the needle passes through the ligamentum flavum and the spinal arachnoid membrane.

If the needle hits bone deep, withdraw back through the ligamentum flavum and redirect needle more caudally. If the patient develops

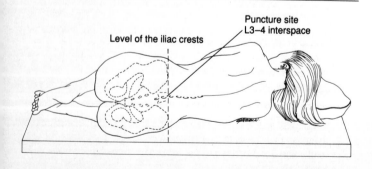

Figure 2–6. Lying position for lumbar puncture. (Reproduced, with permission, from Simon RP et al: *Clinical Neurology.* Appleton & Lange, 1989.)

pain in a leg or buttock, withdraw the needle and redirect it toward the midline and away from the involved side.

When cerebrospinal fluid flows through the needle, discard the first few drops. Then attach the stopcock and manometer to the needle and have the patient slowly relax and uncurl from the fetal position to check the opening CSF pressure (normal 70–180 mm water). (If the patient is seated, either omit measurement of opening pressure or have the patient carefully lie down.)

Remove the manometer and begin collecting samples of CSF in the specimen tubes. Insert the stylet halfway into the shaft of the needle to interrupt the flow of CSF between specimens.

For diagnostic purposes, collect 4 tubes: tube #1 (0.5–1.0 mL); tube #2 (2 mL); tube #3 (2 mL); and tube #4 (1–2 mL) (smaller volumes in children). For therapeutic injections, inject the solution slowly over 30 seconds after first removing at least an equivalent volume of CSF.

If spinal subarachnoid block is suspected, replace the manometer and stopcock and obtain a closing CSF pressure.

Remove the needle and place a small adhesive bandage over the puncture site.

Draw a sample of venous blood to determine comparison serum glucose level.

Have the patient lie *prone* for at least 2 hours after LP to avoid headache.

Possible Complications

Arterial or venous puncture, spinal subdural or epidural hematoma.

Post-lumbar puncture headache.

Infection (meningitis).

Cerebral herniation.

Specimen Handling

Properly dispose of the spinal needle, then gloves (see p 6).

Note the color and clarity of CSF.

Check that each tube is properly labeled.

Send tube #1 for CSF cell count and differential; tube #2 for Gram's stain and culture; tube #3 for CSF protein and glucose determination; and tube #4 for CSF VDRL or other studies (eg, oligoclonal bands or cytology). (***Note:*** If RBC count is high in tube #1, check cell count in tube #4 also.)

8. ARTHROCENTESIS

Indications

To obtain synovial fluid for laboratory analysis.

To drain joint hematoma (hemarthrosis), pus (septic arthritis), or effusion (for symptomatic relief).

To instill local analgesic (eg, lidocaine) and anti-inflammatory agents (eg, corticosteroid) into a joint.

Contraindications

Soft tissue infection over proposed aspiration site.

Severe bleeding diathesis or anticoagulant therapy.

Agitated, uncooperative patient (relative contraindication).

Approach to the Patient

Label each tube with the patient's name and identification number (see p 6).

The major peripheral joints are readily aspirated. Aspiration of the hip and other joints of the axial skeleton is usually performed by an orthopedic surgeon or rheumatologist.

Knee: The knee joint can be entered either medially or laterally (Figure 2–7). The patient should be supine, with the leg fully extended. Apply pressure on the opposite side of the joint from puncture site to assist in directing the needle toward the bulging synovium. From the lateral approach, the needle (held parallel to the bed) is directed medially, just beneath the patella, into the suprapatellar space. From the medial approach, the needle (held parallel to the bed) is introduced between the patella and medial condyle, and advanced upward and laterally, beneath the patella and into the joint space.

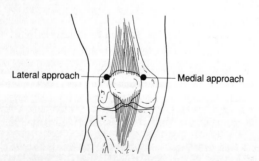

Figure 2–7. Aspiration of the knee joint. (Reproduced, with permission, from: Ho MT et al: *Current Emergency Diagnosis & Treatment*, 3rd ed. Appleton & Lange, 1990.)

Shoulder: The shoulder joint can be aspirated either posteriorly or anteriorly (Figure 2–8). For the posterior approach, have the patient sit backwards in a chair (chest against chair back), placing the arm to be aspirated across the chest with the hand on the opposite shoulder. Insert the needle (held parallel to floor) just under the posterior inferior border of the acromion and advance it, directing it about 30 degrees medially into the joint space (Figure 2–8A). For the anterior approach, have the patient sit in a chair, facing forward, with the arm supported in the lap on a pillow. Insert the needle just medial to the head of the humerus and just below the (palpable) tip of the coracoid process (Figure 2–8B). Direct the needle slightly laterally and superiorly into the scapulohumeral joint space.

Elbow: Be certain to differentiate joint effusion from olecranon bursitis. If effusion is present, have the patient sit with the forearm supported on a table. Insert the needle just below the lateral epicondyle and just proximal to the olecranon process of the radius (Figure 2–9A). Advance the needle medially and slightly proximally into the joint space.

Ankle: The ankle is usually aspirated anteromedially. Have the patient lie supine, with the knee extended and the foot slightly plantar-flexed. Have the patient extend the great toe and identify the extensor hallucis longus tendon. Just lateral to this tendon and just anterior (1 cm) and inferior (1 cm) to the medial malleolus is

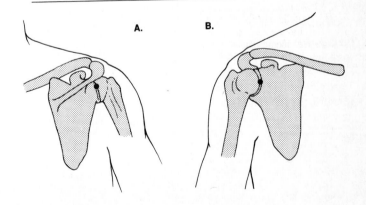

Figure 2–8. A: Posterior approach to aspiration of the shoulder joint. **B:** Anterior approach to aspiration of the shoulder joint. (Reproduced, with permission, from: Ho MT et al: *Current Emergency Diagnosis & Treatment*, 3rd ed. Appleton & Lange, 1990.)

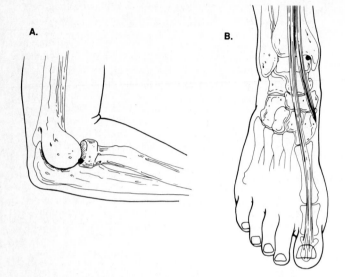

Figure 2–9. A: Aspiration of the elbow. **B:** Aspiration of the ankle joint. (Reproduced, with permission, from: Ho MT et al: *Current Emergency Diagnosis & Treatment*, 3rd ed. Appleton & Lange, 1990.)

a small depression (Figure 2–9B). Insert the needle here and direct it toward the tibiotalar articulation.

Procedural Technique

Stabilize the joint to be aspirated, identify landmarks, and mark the needle insertion point by scratching or indenting skin.

Observe sterile technique (don mask and gloves).

Sterilize the skin around the insertion site with iodine.

Anesthetize the skin over the insertion site with 1% lidocaine, using a 5-mL syringe and a 25- or 27- gauge needle; then anesthetize down to the joint capsule.

Using a 20-gauge needle (larger gauge if fluid is very viscous) and a 10-mL syringe, penetrate the skin at the selected site and advance the needle into the joint space, maintaining constant, gentle suction on the syringe. Stop advancing the needle when joint fluid flows into the syringe.

Remove as much joint fluid as possible.

Withdraw the needle and apply firm pressure over the insertion site for 1–2 minutes. Cover with an adhesive dressing.

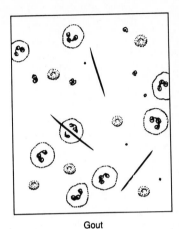
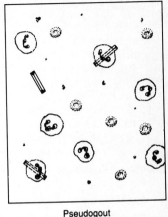

Gout   Pseudogout

Figure 2–10. Examination of synovial fluid for crystals, using a compensated polarized microscope. In gout, crystals are needle-shaped, negatively birefringent, and composed of monosodium urate. In pseudogout, crystals are rhomboidal, positively birefringent, and composed of calcium pyrophosphate dihydrate (CPPD). In both diseases, crystals can be found free-floating or within polymorphonuclear cells.

Possible Complications

Bleeding (hemarthrosis).

Infection (septic arthritis).

Specimen Handling

Fill the tubes completely with synovial fluid and tilt each tube containing anticoagulant or preservative to mix thoroughly.

Properly dispose of the needle, then gloves (see p 6).

Check that each tube is properly labeled. Record the amount of joint (synovial) fluid removed and its color and clarity. Note the fluid viscosity by allowing a drop to fall from the needle (normal fluid has high viscosity and easily forms a thread several inches long). Joint fluid should be sent for: cell count and differential (purple top); glucose (red top); culture and Gram's stain (sterile tube); and microscopic examination for crystals (green top). Figure 2–10 shows typical morphology for gout and pseudogout crystals. If neoplasm (pigmented villonodular synovitis or metastatic disease) is suspected, fluid may be sent for cytology (in a cytology bottle). (See p 238 for guide to interpretation of synovial fluid findings.)

9. BASIC STAINING METHODS

A. Gram's Stain

Preparation of Smear

Obtain a fresh specimen of the material to be stained (eg, sputum) and smear a small amount on a glass slide. Thin smears give the best results (eg, press a sputum sample between two glass slides).

Let the smear air dry before heat fixing, because heating a wet smear will usually distort cells and organisms.

Heat fix the smear by passing the back side of the slide quickly through a Bunsen burner or other flame (no more than 3 or 4 times). The slide should be warm, not hot.

Let the slide cool before staining.

Staining Technique

Put on gloves.

Stain with crystal violet (10 seconds).

Rinse with gently running water (5 seconds).

Flood with Gram's iodine solution (10–30 seconds).

Rinse with gently running water (5 seconds).

Decolorize with acetone-alcohol solution until no more blue color leaches from the slide (5 seconds).

Rinse immediately with water (5 seconds).

Counterstain with safranine red (10 seconds).

Rinse with water (5 seconds).

Let the slide air dry (or carefully blot with filter paper), then examine it under the microscope.

Microscopic Examination

Examine the smear first using the low-power lens for leukocytes and fungi. Screen for the number and color of polymorphonuclear cells (cells should be pink, not blue).

Examine using the high-power oil-immersion lens for microbial forms. Screen for intracellular organisms. Review the slide systematically for (1) fungi (mycelia, then yeast), (2) small gram-negative rods (*Bacteroides*, *Haemophilus*, etc) (3) gram-negative cocci (*Neisseria*, etc), (4) gram-positive rods (*Listeria*, etc), and (5) gram-positive cocci (*Streptococcus*, *Staphylococcus*, etc).

Label positive slides with the patient's name and save them for later review.

Figure 2–11 illustrates typical sputum Gram's stain findings.

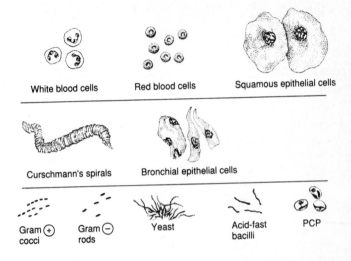

Figure 2–11. Common findings on microscopic examination of the sputum. Most elements can be seen with Gram's stain, except for acid-fast bacilli (Kinyoun stain) and *Pneumocystis Carinii* (PCP) (Giemsa stain). (Modified and reproduced, with permission, from Krupp MA et al: *Physicians's Handbook*, 21st ed. Lange, 1985.)

B. Acid-fast (Kinyoun) Stain

Preparation of Smear

As above for Gram's stain: fix the air-dried thin smear by passing it quickly through a flame (3 or 4 times). Let the smear cool before staining.

Staining Technique

Put on gloves.

Stain with Kinyoun stain (5 minutes).

Rinse with gently running water (5 seconds).

Decolorize with acid/alcohol solution until no more color leaches from the slide (3–4 minutes).

Rinse well with water (5 seconds).

Counterstain with methylene blue (2 minutes).

Rinse thoroughly with water (5 seconds).

Let the slide air dry (do not blot), then examine it under the microscope.

Microscopic Examination

Examine the smear first using the low-power lens for leukocytes (cells should be blue, not pink).

Examine using the high-power oil immersion lens for acid-fast bacilli (AFB appear as bright pink against the blue background). Review the slide systematically for 5 minutes or longer.

Label positive slides with the patient's name and save them for later review.

C. Wright's Stain of Peripheral Blood Smear

Preparation of Smear

Obtain a fresh specimen of blood by pricking the patient's finger with a lancet. If alcohol is used to clean the fingertip, wipe it off with a gauze pad.

Place a single drop of blood on a glass slide. Drop a second glass slide on top and rapidly pull lengthwise to produce a thin smear.

Let the smear air dry. Do not heat-fix.

Staining Technique

Stain with fresh Wright's stain (1 minute).

Gently add an equal amount of water and gently blow on the smear to mix the stain and water. Repeat by adding more water and blowing to mix. Look for formation of a shiny surface scum. Then allow the stain to set (3–4 minutes).

Rinse with gently running water (5 seconds).

Clean the back of the slide with an alcohol pad if necessary.

Microscopic Examination

Examine the smear first using the low-power lens to select a good area for study (red and white cells separated from one another).

Then move to the high-power oil-immersion lens. Review the slide systematically for (1) platelet morphology, (2) white cells (differential types, morphology, toxic granulations and vacuoles, etc), and (3) red cells (size, shape, color, stippling, nucleated, etc).

Label slides with the patient's name and save them for later review.

See Figure 2–12 below for examples of common peripheral blood smear abnormalities.

D. Methylene Blue Stain for Fecal Leukocytes

Preparation of Smear

Place a small amount of mucus (or stool if no mucus is present) on a glass slide. *Note:* This technique is unreliable if the sample is taken from a rectal swab, a dried stool smear, or the center of formed stool.

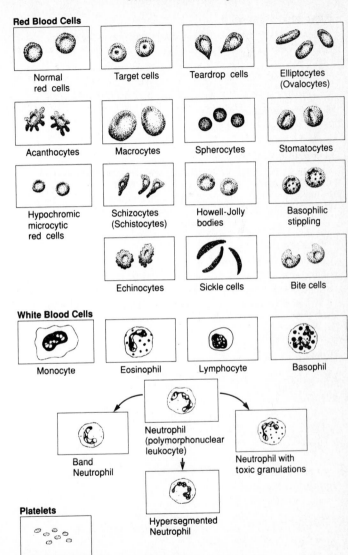

Figure 2–12. Common peripheral blood smear findings.

Staining Technique

Add 2 drops of methylene blue solution. Mix thoroughly.

Place a coverslip over the area to be examined.

Wait 2–3 minutes for cell nuclei to take up the stain.

(Alternatively, you may perform a Wright's stain of dried mucus, using the same technique as for the peripheral blood smear.)

Microscopic Examination

Examine under the microscope, using the high dry, then oil immersion lenses.

Look for leukocytes and bacteria.

Screen for both polymorphonuclear and mononuclear cells (cell nuclei should be blue). Presence of any fecal leukocytes is abnormal and indicates inflammation or disruption of colonic mucosal lining (infectious diarrheal disorders—eg, shigellosis, salmonellosis, invasive *E coli* colitis, amebic colitis, pseudomembranous colitis—ulcerative colitis, Crohn's disease, diverticulitis, or necrotic neoplasm).

Normally, there are many types of bacteria. In children with diarrhea, examine using the high-power oil-immersion lens to exclude staphylococcal enterocolitis (single bacterial coccal form present).

Label positive slides with the patient's name and save them for later review.

E. Tzanck Smear

Preparation of Smear

Use an alcohol pad to gently clean the skin. Wipe the alcohol off with a gauze pad, or let the skin air dry.

Obtain a specimen by removing the top of a blister with a No. 15 scalpel blade, being careful not to disturb its base.

Then gently scrape the blade edge across the exposed floor of the blister. Smear the material adhering to the forward edge of the blade on a glass slide.

Let the smear air dry, or heat-fix.

Staining Technique

Stain with fresh Wright's stain (using the same technique as for peripheral blood smear) or fresh Giemsa stain. If Giemsa stain is used, the specimen must first be fixed to the slide with methyl alcohol for 10–15 minutes.

Clean the back of the slide with an alcohol pad, if necessary.

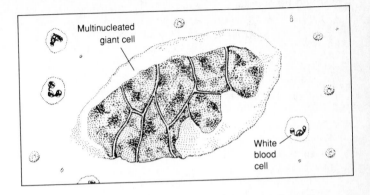

Figure 2–13. Tzanck smear showing a multinucleated giant cell.

Microscopic Examination

Examine the smear first using the low-power lens to select a good area for study.

Then move to the high-power oil-immersion lens. Review the slide for multinucleated giant cells (Figure 2–13) from viral infection of epidermal cells (eg, herpes simplex, varicella-zoster viruses).

Label positive slides with the patient's name and save them for later review.

10. OTHER

A. Urinalysis

Collection and Preparation of Specimen

Obtain a midstream urine specimen from the patient. The sample must be free of skin epithelium or bacteria, secretions, hair, lint, etc.

Examine the specimen while fresh (still warm). Otherwise, bacteria may proliferate, casts and crystals may dissolve, and particulate matter may settle out. (Occasionally, amorphous crystals precipitate out, obscuring formed elements. In cold urine, they are amorphous urate crystals; these may be dissolved by gently rewarming the urine. In alkaline urine, they are amorphous phosphate crystals; these may be dissolved by adding 1 mL of acetic acid.)

Place 10 mL in a tube and centrifuge at 2000–3000 rpm for 3–5 minutes.

Discard the supernatant. Resuspend the sediment in the few drops that remain by gently tilting the tube.

Place a drop on a glass slide, cover it with a coverslip, and examine under the microscope; no stain is needed. If bacterial infection is present, a single drop of methylene blue applied to the edge of the coverslip, or a Gram's stain of an air-dried, heat-fixed specimen, can assist in distinguishing gram-negative rods (eg, *E coli, Proteus, Klebsiella*) from gram-positive cocci (eg, *Enterococcus, Staphylococcus saprophyticus*).

Procedural Technique

While the urine is centrifuging, examine the remainder of the specimen by inspection and reagent strip ("dipstick") testing.

Inspect the specimen for color and clarity. Normally, urine is yellow or light orange. Dark orange urine is caused by phenazopyridine (eg, Pyridium) therapy; red urine, by hemoglobinuria, myoglobinuria, beets, senna, or rifampin therapy; green urine, by *Pseudomonas* infection or iodochlorhydroxyquin or amitriptyline therapy; brown urine, by bilirubinuria or fecal contamination; black urine, by intravascular hemolysis, alkaptonuria, melanoma, or methyldopa therapy; purplish urine, by porphyria; and milky white urine, by pus, chyluria, or amorphous crystals (urates or phosphates). Turbidity of urine is caused by pus, red blood cells, or crystals.

Reagent strips provide information about specific gravity, pH, protein, glucose, ketone, bilirubin, heme, nitrite, and esterase (see Table 2–1 below). Dip a reagent strip in the urine and compare it with the chart on the bottle. Follow the timing instructions carefully. *Note:* Reagent strips cannot be relied on to detect some proteins (eg, globulins, light chains) or sugars (other than glucose).

Record the results.

Microscopic Examination

Examine the area under the coverslip under the low-power and high-dry lenses for cells, casts, crystals, and bacteria. (If a Gram's stain is done, examine under the oil immersion lens.)

Cells may be red cells, white cells, squamous cells, transitional (bladder) epithelial cells, or atypical (tumor) cells. Red cells suggest upper or lower urinary tract infections (cystitis, prostatitis, pyelonephritis), glomerulonephritis, collagen-vascular disease, trauma, renal calculi, tumors, drug reactions, and structural abnormalities (polycystic kidneys). White cells suggest inflammatory processes such as urinary tract infection (most common), collagen vascular disease or interstitial nephritis. Red cell casts are considered pathognomonic of glomerulonephritis; white cell casts, of pyelonephritis; and fatty (lipid) casts, of nephrotic syndrome.

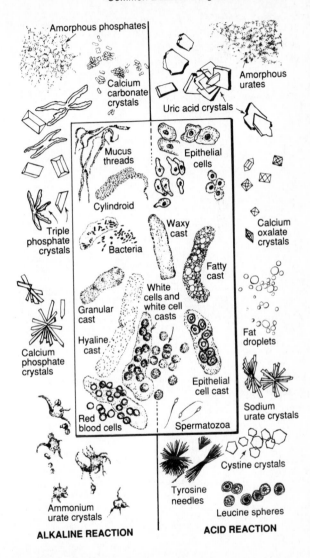

Figure 2–14. Microscopic findings on examination of the urine. (Modified and reproduced, with permission, from: Krupp MA et al: *Physician's Handbook*, 21st ed. Lange, 1985.)

Table 2–1. Components of the urine dipstick.[1]

Test	Expected Values	Lowest Detectable Range	Comments
Specific Gravity	1.003–1.040	1.000–1.030	Highly buffered alkaline urine may yield low specific gravity readings. Moderate proteinuria (100–750 mg/dL) may yield high specific gravity readings. Loss of concentrating or diluting capacity indicates renal dysfunction.
pH	5–9 units	5–8.5 units	Excessive urine on strip may cause protein reagent to run over onto pH area, yielding falsely low pH reading.
Protein	0	15–30 mg/dL albumin	False negative readings can be caused by highly buffered alkaline urine. Reagent more sensitive to albumin than other proteins. A negative result does not rule out the presence of globulins, hemoglobin, Bence Jones proteins or mucoprotein. 1+ = 30 mg/dL 3+ = 300 mg/dL 2+ = 100 mg/dL 4+ ≥ 2000 mg/dL
Glucose	0	75–125 mg/dL	Test is specific for glucose. False-negative results occur with urinary ascorbic acid concentrations ≥ 50 mg/dL and with ketone body levels ≥ 40 mg/dL. Test reagent reactivity also varies with specific gravity and temperature. trace = 100 mg/dL 1 = 1000 mg/dL 1/4 = 250 mg/dL 2 ≥ 2000 mg/dL 1/2 = 500 mg/dL
Ketone	0	5–10 mg/dL acetoacetate	Test does not react with acetone or ß-hydroxybutyric acid. (Trace) false-positive results may occur with high specific gravity/low pH urines, highly pigmented urines, or those containing levodopa metabolites or sulfhydryl-containing compounds. Trace = 5 mg/dL Moderate = 40 mg/dL Small = 15 mg/dL Large = 50–160 mg/dL
Bilirubin	0	0.4–0.8 mg/dL	Indicates hepatitis (conjugated bilirubin). False-negative readings can be caused by ascorbic acid concentrations ≥ 25 mg/dL. Test is less sensitive than Ictotest Reagent tablets.
Blood	0[2]	0.015–0.062 mg/dL hemoglobin	Test equally sensitive to myoglobin and hemoglobin (including both intact erythrocytes and free hemoglobin). False-positive results can be caused by oxidizing contaminants (hypochlorite) and microbial peroxidase (urinary tract infection). Test sensitivity is reduced in urines with high specific gravity, ascorbic acid, or heavy proteinuria.
Nitrite	0	0.06–0.1 mg/dL	Test depends on the conversion of nitrate (derived from the diet) to nitrite by gram-negative bacteria in urine. Test specific for nitrite. False-negative readings can be caused by ascorbic acid.
Leukocytes (esterase)	0[3]	5–15 WBCs/hpf	Indicator of urinary tract infection. Test detects esterases contained in granulocytic leukocytes. Test sensitivity is reduced in urines with high specific gravity, elevated glucose concentrations (≥ 3 g/dL), or presence of cephalexin, cephalothin, tetracycline, or high concentrations of oxalate.

[1] Package insert, revised 8/90. Ames Reagent Strip for N-Multistix SG. Ames Division, Miles Laboratory.
[2] Except in menstruating females
[3] Except in females with vaginitis

The finding on a Gram's stain of unspun, clean, fresh urine of even one bacterium per field under the oil-immersion lens correlates fairly well with bacterial culture colony counts of greater than 100,000 organisms per μL.

(See Table 7–20, p 244, for guide to interpretation of urinalysis, and Figure 2–14, p 33, for guide to microscopic findings in urine.)

B. Vaginal Fluid Wet Preparation

Preparation of Smear

Place a small amount of vaginal discharge on a glass slide.

Staining Technique

Add 2 drops of sterile saline solution.

Place a coverslip over the area to be examined.

Microscopic Examination

Examine under the microscope, using the high-dry lens and a low light source.

Look for motile trichomonads (undulating protozoa propelled by 4 flagella). Look for clue cells (vaginal epithelial cells with large numbers of organisms attached to them, obscuring cell borders), pathognomonic of *Gardnerella vaginalis*-associated vaginosis.

See Figure 2–15 below for an example of a positive wet prep (Trichomonads, clue cells) and p 245 for differential diagnosis of vaginal discharge.

C. Skin or Vaginal Fluid KOH Preparation

Preparation of Smear

Obtain a specimen by using a No. 15 Bard-Parker scalpel blade to scrape scales from the skin lesion onto a glass slide or to remove the top of a vesicle onto the slide. Or place a single drop of vaginal discharge on the slide.

Staining Technique

Place 1–2 drops of potassium hydroxide (10–20%) on top of the specimen on the slide. Drop a coverslip on the area to be examined.

Heat the slide from beneath by a match or Bunsen burner flame until the slide contents begin to bubble.

Clean carbon off the back side of the slide with an alcohol pad, if necessary.

Note: A fishy amine odor upon addition of KOH to a vaginal discharge is typical of bacterial vaginosis caused by *Gardnerella vaginalis*.

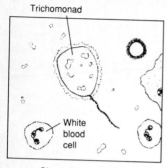

Trichomonad

White blood cell

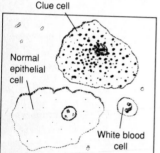

Clue cell

Normal epithelial cell

White blood cell

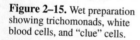

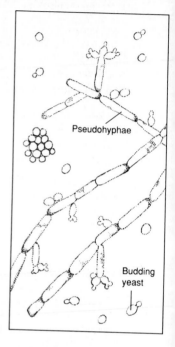

Pseudohyphae

Budding yeast

Figure 2–15. Wet preparation showing trichomonads, white blood cells, and "clue" cells.

Figure 2–16. KOH preparation showing mycelial forms (pseudohyphae) and budding yeast typical of *Candida albicans*.

Microscopic Examination

Examine the smear under the high-dry lens for mycelial forms. Branched, septate hyphae are typical of dermatophytosis (eg, *Trichophyton, Epidermophyton, Microsporum* spp); branched, septate pseudohyphae with or without budding yeast forms are seen with candidiasis (*Candida* spp); and short, curved hyphae plus clumps of spores ("spaghetti and meatballs") are seen with tinea versicolor (*Pityrosporum orbiculare*).

(See Figure 2–16 above for an example of a positive KOH prep.)

D. Pulse Oximetry

Indications

To measure oxygen saturation in a noninvasive and often continuous fashion.

Contraindications

Hypotension, hypothermia, and severe anemia (hemoglobin < 5 g/dL) causes inaccurate readings.

Hyperbilirubinemia, methemoglobinemia, fetal hemoglobinemia, and carboxyhemoglobinemia can falsely elevate oxygen saturation measurements.

Excessive ambient light, simultaneous use of a blood pressure cuff, presence of intravascular dyes (eg, methylene blue), and electrical interference (eg, MRI scanners, electrosurgery) can also cause erroneous readings.

Approach to the Patient

The patient should be positioned close to the pulse oximeter and should hold the probe site still. The sampling area should have good circulation and be free of skin irritation.

Procedural Technique

Plug the pulse oximeter into a grounded AC power outlet or make sure there is sufficient battery power available. Turn the oximeter on and wait until self-calibration is complete.

Select the probe to be used and connect it to the pulse oximeter. The probe consists of a light source (a red light emitting device [LED] in most cases) and a photodetector. Probes are available for the ear, finger, and, in neonates, the foot, ankle, palm, calf and forearm.

Attach the probe to the patient after using an alcohol swab to cleanse the surrounding skin. Some probes come with double-sided adhesive disks which improve probe signal.

Watch the waveform and pulse indicators to assess the quality of the signal. Readjust if a poor signal is present.

Set alarm warnings on the device.

Check the probe site at least every four hours. Care should be taken not to apply tension to the probe cables.

Possible Complications

Allergic reaction to adhesives.

Comments

Because of the curvilinear nature of the oxygen-hemoglobin dissociation curve, oxygen saturation (SaO_2) is not directly proportional to oxygen partial pressure (PaO_2). Therefore, a relatively small change in oxygen saturation from 94% to 83% can represent a large change in PaO_2 from 80 to 50 mm Hg. In addition, the dissociation curve varies markedly from patient to patient and with pH, temperature, and altitude. To ensure accurate assessment of oxygenation, one should correlate pulse oximetry with arterial blood gas analysis.

3 Common Laboratory Tests: Selection & Interpretation

HOW TO USE THIS SECTION

This section contains information about commonly used laboratory tests. It includes most of the blood, urine, and cerebrospinal fluid tests found in this book, with the exception of drug levels (Chapter 4). Entries are in tabular form and are arranged alphabetically.

Test/Reference Range/Collection

This first column begins with the common test name, the fluid the specimen is obtained from, and any test name abbreviation (in parentheses).

Below this is the reference range for each test. The first entry is in conventional units and the second entry (in brackets) is in SI units (Système International d'Unités). Any panic values for a particular test will be placed here after the word "Panic." The reference ranges provided are from several large medical centers. Consult your own clinical laboratory for the reference ranges used in your institution.

This column also shows which tube to use for collecting blood or other body fluid, how much the test costs, and how to collect the specimen. Listed below are the common collection tubes and their contents:

Tube Color	Tube Contents	Typically Used in
Lavender	EDTA	Complete blood count
Marbled	Serum separator	Serum chemistry tests
Red	None	Blood banking (serum)
Blue	Citrate	Coagulation studies
Green	Heparin	Plasma studies
Yellow	Acid citrate	HLA typing
Navy	Trace metal free	Trace metals (eg, lead)

The scale used for the cost of each test is:

Approximate Cost	Symbol Used in Tables
$1–20	$
$21–50	$$
$51–100	$$$
> $100	$$$$

Physiologic Basis

This column contains physiologic information about the substance being tested. Information on classification and biologic importance, as well as interactions with other biologic substances and processes, are included.

Interpretation (sensitivity)

This column lists clinical conditions that affect the substance being tested. Generally, conditions with higher prevalence will be listed first. When the sensitivity of the test for a particular disease is known, it will follow the disease name in parentheses, eg, "rheumatoid arthritis (83%)". Some of the common drugs that can affect the test substance in vivo will also be included in this column.

Comments

This column contains general information pertinent to the use and interpretation of the test substance and important in vitro interferences with the test procedure. Appropriate general references are also listed.

Test Name

In the last column the test name is placed perpendicularly to the rest of the table to allow for quick referencing.

Reference

Young DS: Implementation of SI units for clinical laboratory data. Ann Intern Med 1987;106:114.

Test/Range/Collection	Physiologic Basis	Interpretation (sensitivity)	Comments
ABO grouping, serum and red cells (ABO) Red and lavender $ Properly identified and labeled blood specimens are critical.	The 4 blood groups A, B, O, and AB are determined by the presence or absence of antigens A and B or their absence (O) on a patient's red blood cells. Antibodies are present in serum in which red cells lack antigen.	In the US white population, 45% are type O, 40% A, 11% B, 4% AB. In the African-American population, 49% are type O, 27% A, 20% B, 4% AB. In the US Asian population, 40% are type O, 28% A, 27% B, 5% AB. In the Native American population, 79% are type 0, 16% A, 4% B, <1% AB.	For both blood donors and recipients, routine ABO grouping includes both red cell and serum testing, as checks on each other. Tube testing is as follows: patient's red cells are tested with anti-A and anti-B for the presence or absence of agglutination (forward or cell grouping) and patient's serum is tested against known A and B cells (reverse or serum grouping). Ref: *Technical Manual of the American Association of Blood Banks,* 10th ed. American Association of Blood Banks, 1990.
Acetaminophen, serum (Tylenol) 10–20 mg/L [66–132 µmol/L] ***Panic:*** >50 mg/L Marbled $$ For suspected overdose, draw 2 samples at least 4 hours apart, at least 4 hours after ingestion. Note time of ingestion, if known. Order test stat.	In overdose, liver and renal toxicity is produced by the hydroxylated metabolite if it is not conjugated with glutathione in the liver.	**Increased in:** Acetaminophen overdose. Interpretation of serum acetaminophen level depends on time since ingestion. Levels drawn < 4 hours after ingestion cannot be interpreted since the drug is still in the absorption and distribution phase. Use nomogram (Figure 9–1, p 260) to evaluate possible toxicity. Levels > 150 mg/dL at 4 hours or > 50 mg/dL at 12 hours after ingestion suggest toxicity.	Do not delay acetylcysteine (Mucomyst) treatment (140 mg/kg orally) if stat levels are unavailable. Ref: Lancet 1976;2:109. Ref: Lancet 1971;1:519. Ref: Pediatrics 1975;55:871.

	Acetoacetate			Acid phosphatase
Test/Range/Collection	Physiologic Basis	Interpretation (sensitivity)	Comments	
Acetoacetate, serum or urine 0 mg/dL [µmol/L] Marbled or urine container $ Urine sample should be fresh.	Acetoacetate, acetone, and β-hydroxybutyrate contribute to ketoacidosis when oxidative hepatic metabolism of fatty acids is impaired. Proportions in serum vary but are generally 20% acetoacetate, 78% β-hydroxybutyrate, and 2% acetone.	**Present in:** Diabetic ketoacidosis, alcoholic ketoacidosis, prolonged fasting, severe carbohydrate restriction with normal fat intake.	Nitroprusside test is semiquantitative; it detects acetoacetate and is sensitive down to 5–10 mg/dL. Trace = 5 mg/dL, small = 15 mg/dL, moderate = 40 mg/dL, large = 80 mg/dL [1 mg/dL =100 µmol/L]. β-hydroxybutyrate is not a ketone and is not detected by the nitroprusside test. Acetone is not reliably detected by this method. Failure of test to detect β-hydroxybutyrate in ketoacidosis may produce a seemingly paradoxical increase in ketones with clinical improvement as nondetectable β-hydroxybutyrate is replaced by detectable acetoacetate. Ref: Br Med J 1972;2:565.	
Acid phosphatase (prostatic), serum 0.1–0.9 IU/L [< 15 nkat/L] (method-dependent) Marbled $$ Rapid loss of enzyme activity unless kept at pH 5–6 and analyzed promptly.	Acid phosphatases are present in high concentration in the prostate gland, erythrocytes, platelets, liver, and spleen.	**Increased in:** Carcinoma of prostate (91% stage D, 18% stage A), prostate palpation or surgery, benign prostatic hypertrophy, Gaucher's disease.	Test has been largely replaced by prostate-specific antigen, which is much more sensitive (see p 118). Only use is in monitoring prostate cancer patients on hormone therapy. It is not a good screening test. Ref: JAMA 1985;253:665. Ref: Am J Clin Pathol 1985;84:334.	

		ACTH	**ALT**
Adrenocorticotropic hormone, plasma (ACTH) 20–100 pg/mL [4–22 pmol/L] Heparinized plastic container $$$$ Send promptly to laboratory on ice. ACTH is unstable in plasma, is inactivated at room temperature, and adheres strongly to glass. Avoid all contact with glass.	Pituitary ACTH (release stimulated by hypothalamic corticotropin-releasing factor) stimulates cortisol release from the adrenal gland. There is feedback regulation of the system by cortisol. ACTH is secreted episodically and shows circadian variation, with highest levels at 6:00–8:00 AM; lowest levels at 9:00–10:00 PM.	**Increased in:** Pituitary (40–200 pg/mL) and ectopic (200–71,000 pg/mL) Cushing's syndrome, primary adrenal insufficiency (> 250 pg/mL), adrenogenital syndrome with impaired cortisol production. **Decreased in:** Adrenal Cushing's syndrome (< 20 pg/mL), pituitary ACTH (secondary adrenal) insufficiency (< 50 pg/mL).	ACTH levels (RIA) can only be interpreted when measured with cortisol after standardized stimulation or suppression tests (see Adrenocortical insufficiency algorithm, p 250, and Cushing's syndrome algorithm, p 252). Ref: Br Med J 1971;1:374.
Alanine aminotransferase, serum (ALT, SGPT, GPT) 0–35 U/L [0–0.58 μkat/L] (laboratory-specific) Marbled $	Intracellular enzyme involved in amino acid metabolism. Present in large concentrations in liver, kidney; in smaller amounts, in skeletal muscle and heart. Released with tissue damage.	**Increased in:** Acute viral hepatitis (ALT > AST), biliary tract obstruction (cholangitis, choledocholithiasis), alcoholic hepatitis and cirrhosis (AST > ALT), liver abscess, metastatic or primary liver cancer; right heart failure, ischemia or hypoxia, injury to liver ("shock liver"), extensive trauma. Drugs that cause cholestasis or hepatotoxicity. **Decreased in:** Pyridoxine (vitamin B_6) deficiency.	ALT screening of donor blood is used in blood banks to exclude non-A, non-B hepatitis. Ref: Arch Intern Med 1991;151:260. Ref: Clin Biochem 1990;23:375.

Test/Range/Collection	Physiologic Basis	Interpretation (sensitivity)	Comments
Albumin, serum 3.4–4.7 g/dL [34–47 g/L] Marbled $	Major component of plasma proteins; influenced by nutritional state, hepatic function, renal function, and various diseases.	**Increased in:** Dehydration, shock, hemoconcentration. **Decreased in:** Decreased hepatic synthesis (chronic liver disease, malnutrition, malabsorption, malignancy, congenital analbuminemia [rare]). Increased losses (nephrotic syndrome, burns, trauma, hemorrhage with fluid replacement, fistulas, enteropathy, acute or chronic glomerulonephritis). Hemodilution (pregnancy, CHF). Drugs: estrogens.	Serum albumin gives an indication of severity in chronic liver disease. Useful in nutritional assessment if there is no impairment in production or increased loss of albumin. Ref: Ann Clin Biochem 1985;22:565.
Aldosterone, plasma *Salt-loaded* (120 meq Na$^+$/d): Supine: 3–10 Upright: 5–30 ng/dL *Salt-depleted* (10 meq Na$^+$/d): Supine: 12–36 Upright: 17–137 ng/dL [1 ng/dL = 27.7 pmol/L] Lavender or green $$$$ Early AM fasting specimen. Separate immediately and freeze.	Aldosterone is the major mineralocorticoid hormone and is a major regulator of extracellular volume and serum potassium concentration. For evaluation of hyperaldosteronism (associated with hypertension and hypokalemia), patients should be salt-loaded and recumbent when specimen is drawn. For evaluation of hypoaldosteronism (associated with hyperkalemia), patients should be salt-depleted and upright when specimen is drawn.	**Increased in:** Primary hyperaldosteronism (72%). **Decreased in:** Primary or secondary hypoaldosteronism.	Testing for hyperaldosteronism and hypoaldosteronism must be done using specific protocols, and results must be interpreted based on reference values from the laboratory performing the test. 24-hour urinary excretion of aldosterone is the most sensitive test for hyperaldosteronism (see Aldosterone, urine, below). The significance of an elevated plasma aldosterone level is difficult to interpret without simultaneous determination of plasma renin activity (PRA). In primary aldosteronism, plasma aldosterone is usually elevated while PRA is low; in secondary hyperaldosteronism, both plasma aldosterone and PRA are usually elevated. Ref: Mayo Clin Proc 1990;65:96. Ref: Med Clin N Am 1988;72(5):1117. Ref: Am J Med 1983;74:641.

	Aldosterone, urine			Alkaline phosphatase
Aldosterone, urine *Salt-loaded* (120 meq Na+/d for 3–4 days): 1.5–12.5 µg/24 h *Salt-depleted* (20 meq Na+/d for 3–4 days): 18–85 µg/24 h [1 µg/24 h = 2.77 nmol/d] Bottle containing boric acid $$$$	Secretion of aldosterone is controlled by the renin-angiotensin system. Renin (synthesized and stored in juxtaglomerular cells of kidney) is released in response to both decreased perfusion pressure at the juxtaglomerular apparatus and negative sodium balance. Renin then hydrolyses angiotensinogen to angiotensin I, which is converted to angiotensin II, which then stimulates the adrenal to produce aldosterone. To evaluate hyperaldosteronism, patient is salt-loaded and recumbent. Obtain 24-hour urine for aldosterone (and sodium to check that sodium excretion > 250 meq/day). To evaluate hypoaldosteronism, patient is salt-depleted and upright; check patient for hypotension before 24-hour urine collected.	**Increased in:** Primary and secondary hyperaldosteronism, some patients with essential hypertension. **Decreased in:** Primary hypoaldosteronism (eg, 18-hydroxylase deficiency), secondary hypoaldosteronism (hyporeninemic hypoaldosteronism).	Urinary aldosterone is the most sensitive test for primary hyperaldosteronism. Levels > 14 µg/24 h after 3 days of salt-loading have a 96% sensitivity and 93% specificity for primary hyperaldosteronism. Only 7% of patients with essential hypertension have urinary aldosterone levels > 14 µg/24 h after salt-loading. Neither serum potassium nor plasma renin activity (PRA) is a satisfactory screening test for hyperaldosteronism. Hypokalemia is present in only 73% of patients with hyperaldosteronism on a normal sodium diet, and in 86% after salt loading. Suppressed PRA has only a 64% sensitivity and 83% specificity for hyperaldosteronism. Ref: Mayo Clin Proc 1990;65:96. Ref: Med Clin N Am 1988;72(5):1117. Ref: Am J Med 1983;74:641.
Alkaline phosphatase, serum 41–133 IU/L [0.7–2.2 µkat/L] (method- and age-dependent) Marbled $	Alkaline phosphatases are found in liver, bone, intestine, and placenta.	**Increased in:** Obstructive hepatobiliary disease, bone disease (physiologic bone growth, Paget's disease, osteomalacia, osteogenic sarcoma, bone metastases), hyperparathyroidism, rickets, benign familial hyperphosphatasemia, pregnancy (3rd trimester), GI disease (perforated ulcer or bowel infarct), hepatotoxic drugs. **Decreased in:** Hypophosphatasia.	Normal in osteoporosis. Alkaline phosphatase isoenzyme separation by electrophoresis or differential heat inactivation is unreliable. Use γ-glutamyl transpeptidase (GGT), which increases in hepatobiliary disease but not in bone disease, to infer origin of increased alkaline phosphatase (ie, liver or bone). Ref: Arch Pathol Lab Med 1978;102:509.

Test/Range/Collection	Physiologic Basis	Interpretation (sensitivity)	Comments
Amebic serology, serum < 1:64 titer Marbled $$	Test for presence of *Entamoeba histolytica* by detection of antibodies which develop 2–4 weeks after infection. Tissue invasion by the organism may be necessary for antibody production.	**Increased in:** Current or past infection with *E histolytica.* Amebic abscess (91%), amebic dysentery (84%), asymptomatic cyst carriers (9%), patients with other diseases and healthy people (2%).	In some endemic areas, as many as 44% of those tested have positive serologies. Precipitin or indirect hemagglutination (IHA) tests are available. Ref: N Engl J Med 1978;298:262.
Ammonia, plasma (NH_3) 18–60 µg/dL [11–35 µmol/L] Green $$ Separate plasma from cells immediately. Avoid hemolysis. Analyze immediately. Place on ice.	Ammonia is liberated by bacteria in the large intestine or by protein metabolism and is rapidly converted to urea in liver. In liver disease or portal-systemic shunting, the blood ammonia concentration increases.	**Increased in:** Hepatic insufficiency (especially if protein consumption is high or if there is GI bleeding), fulminant hepatic failure, Reye's syndrome, portacaval shunting, cirrhosis, urea cycle metabolic defects, and organic acidemias. Drugs: diuretics, acetazolamide, asparaginase, others. Spuriously increased by any ammonia-containing detergent on laboratory glassware. **Decreased in:** Decreased production by gut bacteria (kanamycin, neomycin). Decreased gut absorption (lactulose).	Correlates poorly with degree of hepatic encephalopathy. Test not useful in adults with known liver disease. Test is not as useful as CSF glutamine (see p 85). Ref: Clin Chem 1984;30:906.

	Amylase	ACE
Amylase, serum 20–110 U/L [0.33–1.83 μkat/L] (laboratory-specific) Marbled $	Amylase hydrolyzes complex carbohydrates. Serum amylase is derived primarily from pancreas and salivary glands and is increased with inflammation or obstruction of these glands. Other tissues have some amylase activity, including ovaries, small and large intestine, and skeletal muscle.	**Increased in:** Acute pancreatitis (70–95%), pancreatic pseudocyst, pancreatic duct obstruction (cholecystitis, choledocholithiasis, pancreatic carcinoma, stone, stricture, duct sphincter spasm), bowel obstruction and infarction, mumps, parotitis, diabetic ketoacidosis, penetrating peptic ulcer, peritonitis, ruptured ectopic pregnancy, macroamylasemia. Drugs: azathioprine, hydrochlorothiazide. **Decreased in:** Pancreatic insufficiency, cystic fibrosis. Usually normal or low in chronic pancreatitis.	Macroamylasemia is indicated by high serum but low urine amylase. Amylase/creatinine clearance ratio = $$\frac{\text{urine amylase / serum amylase}}{\text{urine creatinine / serum creatinine}} \times 100\%$$ = 1–4%. This ratio was once proposed as a diagnostic test for acute pancreatitis. However, it has been discredited except in the diagnosis of macroamylasemia. Amylase isoenzymes are not of practical use because of technical problems. Ref: Mayo Clin Proc 1979;54:428.
Angiotensin-converting enzyme, serum (ACE) 12–35 U/L [< 590 nkat/L] (method-dependent) Marbled $$	ACE is a dipeptidyl carboxypeptidase that converts angiotensin I to the vasopressor, angiotensin II. ACE is normally present in the kidneys and other peripheral tissues. In granulomatous disease, ACE levels arise from epithelioid cells within granulomas.	**Increased in:** Sarcoidosis (65%), hyperthyroidism, acute hepatitis, primary biliary cirrhosis, diabetes, multiple myeloma, osteoarthritis, amyloidosis, Gaucher's disease, pneumoconiosis, histoplasmosis, miliary tuberculosis. Drugs: dexamethasone. **Decreased in:** Renal disease, obstructive pulmonary disease, hypothyroidism.	Test is not useful as a screening test for sarcoidosis (low sensitivity). Specificity is compromised by positive tests in diseases more common than sarcoidosis. Some advocate measurement of ACE to follow disease activity in sarcoidosis. Ref: JAMA 1979;242:439. Ref: J Clin Pathol 1983;36:938.

	Anti-ds-DNA	Antibody screen

Test/Range/Collection	Physiologic Basis	Interpretation (sensitivity)	Comments
Anti-double-stranded-DNA antibody, serum (ds-DNA) < 1:10 titer Marbled $$	IgG or IgM antibodies directed against host double-stranded DNA.	**Increased in:** Systemic lupus erythematosus (60–70%, 95% specificity). **Not increased in:** Drug-induced lupus.	High titers are seen only in SLE. Titers of anti-ds-DNA correlate well with disease activity and with occurrence of glomerulonephritis. (See also Autoantibodies table, p 226.) Ref: Clin Immunol Immunopath 1988; 47:121. Ref: West J Med 1987;147:210.
Antibody screen, serum Red $ Properly identified and labeled blood specimens are critical.	Detects antibodies to non-ABO red blood cell antigens in recipient's serum, using reagent red cells selected to possess antigens against which common antibodies can be produced. Further identification of the specificity of any antibody detected (using panels of red cells of known antigenicity) makes it possible to test donor blood for the absence of the corresponding antigen.	**Positive in:** Presence of alloantibody, autoantibody.	In practice, a type and screen (ABO and Rh grouping and antibody screen) is adequate workup for patients undergoing operative procedures unlikely to require transfusion. A negative antibody screen implies that a recipient can receive type-specific (ABO-Rh identical) blood with minimal risk. Ref: *Technical Manual of the American Association of Blood Banks*, 10th ed. American Association of Blood Banks, 1990.

Antidiuretic hormone		
Antidiuretic hormone, plasma (ADH) If serum osmolality > 290 mosm/kg H_2O: 2–12 pg/mL If serum osmolality < 290 mosm/kg H_2O: < 2 pg/mL Lavender $$$$ Draw in 2 chilled tubes and deliver to lab on ice. Specimen for osmolality must be drawn at same time.	Antidiuretic hormone (vasopressin) is a hormone secreted from the posterior pituitary that acts on the distal nephron to conserve water and regulate the tonicity of body fluids. Water deprivation provides both an osmotic and a volume stimulus for ADH release by increasing plasma osmolality and decreasing plasma volume. Water administration lowers plasma osmolality and expands blood volume, inhibiting the release of ADH by the osmoreceptor and the atrial volume receptor mechanisms.	**Increased in:** Nephrogenic diabetes insipidus, syndrome of inappropriate antidiuretic hormone (SIADH). Drugs: nicotine, morphine, chlorpropamide, clofibrate, cyclophosphamide. **Normal relative to plasma osmolality in:** Primary polydipsia. **Decreased in:** Central (neurogenic) diabetes insipidus. Drugs: ethanol, phenytoin.	Test very rarely indicated. Measurement of serum and urine osmolality usually suffice. Test not indicated in diagnosis of SIADH. Patients with SIADH show decreased plasma sodium and decreased plasma osmolality, usually with high urine osmolality relative to plasma. These findings in a normovolemic patient with normal thyroid and adrenal function are sufficient to make the diagnosis of SIADH without measuring ADH itself. Ref: N Engl J Med 1981;305:1539.

Test/Range/Collection	Physiologic Basis	Interpretation (sensitivity)	Comments
		Antiglobulin test, direct	**Antiglobulin test, indirect**
Antiglobulin test, direct, red cells (Direct Coombs, DAT) Negative Lavender or red $ Blood anticoagulated with EDTA is used to prevent in vitro uptake of complement components. A red top tube may be used, if necessary.	Direct antiglobulin test demonstrates in vivo coating of washed red cells with globulins, in particular IgG and C3d. Washed red cells are tested directly with antihuman globulin reagent. DAT is positive (shows agglutination) immediately when IgG coats red cells. Complement or IgA coating may only be demonstrated after incubation at room temperature.	**Positive in:** Autoimmune hemolytic anemia, hemolytic disease of the newborn, alloimmune reactions to recently transfused cells, and drug-induced hemolysis. Drugs: cephalosporins, levodopa, methadone, methyldopa, penicillin, quinidine, phenacetin.	A positive DAT implies in vivo red cell coating by immunoglobulins or complement. Such red cell coating may or may not be associated with immune hemolytic anemia. Polyspecific and anti-IgG reagents detect approximately 500 molecules of IgG per red cell, but autoimmune hemolytic anemia has been reported with IgG coating below this level. 10% of hospital patients have a positive DAT without clinical manifestations of immune-mediated hemolysis. A false-positive DAT is often seen in patients with hypergammaglobulinemia. Ref: *Technical Manual of the American Association of Blood Banks*, 10th ed. American Association of Blood Banks, 1990.
Antiglobulin test, indirect, serum (Indirect Coombs) Negative Red $	Demonstrates presence in patient's serum of unexpected antibody to ABO and Rh-compatible red blood cells. First, the patient's serum is incubated in vitro with reagent red cells and washed to remove unbound globulins. Then antihuman globulin (AHG, Coombs) reagent is added. Agglutination of red cells indicates that serum contains antibodies to antigens present on the reagent red cells.	**Positive in:** Presence of alloantibody or autoantibody. Drugs: methyldopa.	The technique is used in antibody detection and identification and in the major cross-match prior to transfusion (see Type and cross-match, p 137). Ref: *Technical Manual of the American Association of Blood Banks*, 10th ed. American Association of Blood Banks, 1990.

	Antimitochondrial antibody	Antinuclear antibody
Antimitochondrial antibody, serum Negative Marbled $$	Qualitative measure of antibodies against hepatic mitochondria. Rabbit hepatocytes are incubated first with serum and then (after washing) with a fluorescein-tagged antibody to human immunoglobulin. Hepatocytes are then viewed for presence of cytoplasmic staining.	**Increased in:** Primary biliary cirrhosis (87–98%), chronic active hepatitis (25–28%); lower titers in viral hepatitis, infectious mononucleosis, neoplasms, cryptogenic cirrhosis (25–30%).	Primarily used to distinguish primary biliary cirrhosis (antibody present) from extrahepatic biliary obstruction (antibody absent). Ref: Hepatology 1986;6:381. Ref: Acta Med Scand 1986;220:241.
Antinuclear antibody (ANA), serum < 1:20 Marbled $$	Heterogeneous antibodies to nuclear antigens (DNA and RNA, histone and nonhistone proteins). Antinuclear antibody is measured in serum by layering the patient's serum over human epithelial cells and detecting the antibody with fluorescein-conjugated polyvalent antihuman immunoglobulin.	**Elevated in:** Patients over age 65 (35–75%, usually in low titers), systemic lupus erythematosus (98%), drug-induced lupus (100%), Sjögren's syndrome (80%), rheumatoid arthritis (30–50%), scleroderma (60%), mixed connective tissue disease (100%), Felty's syndrome, mononucleosis, hepatic or biliary cirrhosis, hepatitis, leukemia, myasthenia gravis, dermatomyositis, polymyositis, chronic renal failure.	A negative ANA test does not completely rule out SLE, but alternative diagnoses should be considered. Pattern of ANA staining may give some clues to diagnoses, but since the pattern also changes with serum dilution, it is not routinely reported. Only the rim (peripheral) pattern is highly specific (for SLE). Not useful as a screening test. Should be used only when there is clinical evidence of a connective tissue disease. Ref: Ann Intern Med 1981;95:333. Ref: West J Med 1987;147:210.

Test/Range/Collection	Physiologic Basis	Interpretation (sensitivity)	Comments
Antistreptolysin O titer, serum (ASO) < 5 years: < 85 5–19 years: < 170 Adults: < 85 Todd units (laboratory-specific) Marbled $$	Detects the presence of antibody to the antigen streptolysin O produced by group A streptococci. Streptococcal antibodies appear about 2 weeks after infection. Titer rises for 4–6 weeks and may remain elevated for 6 months to 1 year. Test is based on the neutralization of hemolytic activity of streptolysin O by antistreptolysin O antibodies in serum.	**Increased in:** Recent infection with group A beta-hemolytic streptococci: scarlet fever, erysipelas, streptococcal pharyngitis/tonsillitis (40–50%), rheumatic fever (80–85%), poststreptococcal glomerulonephritis. Some collagen–vascular diseases. Certain serum lipoproteins, bacterial growth products, or oxidized streptolysin O may result in inhibition of hemolysis and thus cause false-positive results.	Standardization of (Todd) units may vary significantly from laboratory to laboratory. ASO titers are not useful in management of acute streptococcal pharyngitis. In patients with rheumatic fever, test may be a more reliable indicator of recent streptococcal infection than throat culture. An increasing titer is more suggestive of acute streptococcal infection than a single elevated level. Even with severe infection, ASO titers will rise in only 70–80% of patients. Ref: N Engl J Med 1970;282:23,78.
Antithrombin III, plasma (AT III) 84–123% (qualitative) 22–39 mg/dL (quantitative) Blue $$ Transport to lab on ice. Plasma must be separated and frozen in a polypropylene tube within 2 hours.	Antithrombin III is a serine protease inhibitor that protects against thrombus formation by inhibiting thrombin and factors IXa, Xa, XIa, XIIa, plasmin, and kallikrein. It accounts for 70–90% of the anticoagulant activity of human plasma. Its activity is enhanced 100-fold by heparin. There are 2 types of assay: functional (qualitative) and immunologic (quantitative). Since the immunologic assay cannot rule out functional AT III deficiency, a functional assay should be ordered first. Functional assays test AT III activity in inhibiting thrombin. Given an abnormal functional assay, the quantitative immunologic test indicates whether there is decreased synthesis of AT III or intact synthesis of a dysfunctional protein.	**Increased by:** Oral anticoagulants. **Decreased in:** Congenital and acquired AT III deficiency (renal disease, chronic liver disease), oral contraceptive use, chronic disseminated intravascular coagulation, acute venous thrombosis (consumption), and heparin therapy.	Replacement AT III therapy is not available in the USA. Congenital and acquired AT III deficiency results in a hypercoagulable state, venous thromboembolism, and heparin resistance. Congenital AT III deficiency is present in 1:2000–1:5000 people and is autosomal codominant. Heterozygotes have AT III levels 20–60% of normal. Ref: Semin Thromb Hemost 1982;8:276.

	α_1-antitrypsin	AST
α_1-Antitrypsin, serum 110–270 mg/dL [1.1–2.7 g/L] Marbled $$	α_1-Antitrypsin is an α_1 globulin glycoprotein serine protease inhibitor (Pi), whose deficiency leads to excessive trypsin activity and panacinar emphysema in adults or liver disease in children (seen as ZZ and SZ phenotypes). Cirrhosis of the liver and liver cancer in adults are also associated with the Pi Z phenotype.	**Increased in:** Inflammation, infection, rheumatic disease, malignancy, and pregnancy because it is an acute phase reactant. **Decreased in:** Congenital α_1-antitrypsin deficiency, nephrotic syndrome.	Smoking is a much more common cause of chronic obstructive pulmonary disease in adults than is α_1-antitrypsin deficiency. Ref: N Engl J Med 1978;299:1045. Ref: N Engl J Med 1978;299:1099.
Aspartate aminotransferase, serum (AST, SGOT, GOT) 0–35 IU/L [0–0.58 µkat/L] (laboratory-specific) Marbled $	Intracellular enzyme involved in amino acid metabolism. Present in large concentrations in liver, skeletal muscle, brain, red cells, and heart. Released into the bloodstream when tissue is damaged.	**Increased in:** Acute viral hepatitis (ALT > AST), biliary tract obstruction (cholangitis, choledocholithiasis), mononucleosis, alcoholic hepatitis and cirrhosis (AST > ALT), liver abscess, metastatic or primary liver cancer; myocardial infarction, myopathies, muscular dystrophy, dermatomyositis, rhabdomyolysis, ischemic injury to liver ("shock liver") or hypoxia. Hepatotoxic drugs (eg, isoniazid). **Decreased in:** Pyridoxine (vitamin B_6) deficiency.	Test is not indicated for diagnosis of myocardial infarction. Ref: Enzyme 1989;41:112. Ref: Clin Biochem 1990;23:375. Ref: Ann Intern Med 1986;105:221.

Note: The column header "α_1-antitrypsin" spans the first three data columns and "AST" spans the rightmost comments column in the original layout.

Test/Range/Collection	Physiologic Basis	Interpretation (sensitivity)	Comments
Bilirubin, serum 0.1–1.2 mg/dL [2–21 µmol/L] *Direct* (conjugated to glucuronide) bilirubin: 0.1–0.4 mg/dL [< 7 µmol/L]; *Indirect* (unconjugated) bilirubin: 0.2–0.7 mg/dL [< 12 µmol/L] Marbled $$	Bilirubin, a product of hemoglobin metabolism, is conjugated in the liver to mono- and diglucuronides and excreted in bile. Some conjugated bilirubin is bound to serum albumin, so-called D (delta) bilirubin. Elevated serum bilirubin occurs in liver disease, biliary obstruction, or hemolysis.	**Increased in:** Acute or chronic hepatitis, cirrhosis, biliary tract obstruction, toxic hepatitis, congenital liver enzyme abnormalities (Dubin-Johnson, Rotor's, Gilbert's, Crigler-Najjar syndromes), fasting, hemolytic disorders. Hepatotoxic drugs.	Assay of total bilirubin includes conjugated (direct) and unconjugated (indirect) bilirubin plus delta bilirubin (conjugated bilirubin bound to albumin). It is usually clinically unnecessary to fractionate total bilirubin. The diazo reaction is unreliable by the diazo reaction and may underestimate unconjugated bilirubin. Only conjugated bilirubin appears in the urine, and it is indicative of liver disease; hemolysis is associated with increased unconjugated bilirubin. Persistence of delta bilirubin in serum in resolving liver disease means that total bilirubin does not effectively indicate the time course of resolution. Ref: Gastroenterology 1987;92:309. Ref: Blood 1981;57:983.
Bleeding time 2–10 minutes $$ Test done by laboratory personnel. Simplate (presterilized device with spring-loaded blade) used to make single cut 1 mm deep and 6 mm long on dorsal aspect of forearm after inflation of sphygmomanometer to 40 mm Hg. Filter paper is used to absorb blood from wound margins every 30 seconds, and time to cessation of bleeding is noted.	This is a test of platelet function, not a test of coagulation factors.	**Increased in:** Platelet disorders, thrombocytopenia, Bernard-Soulier syndrome, thrombasthenia. Also elevated in some forms of von Willebrand's disease, which is a disorder of factor VIII coagulant activity and not primarily a platelet disorder. Drugs: aspirin and other preparations containing aspirin.	Test is useful as a screening test (with aspirin challenge) for diagnosis of von Willebrand's disease and platelet disorders. Test adds no clinically useful information to the prediction of clinically significant bleeding beyond that obtained from the history, physical examination, and other laboratory tests—platelet count, blood urea nitrogen (BUN), prothrombin time (PT), and partial thromboplastin time (PTT). Ref: Semin Thromb Hemost 1990;16:1.

	BUN	*Brucella* serology
Blood urea nitrogen (BUN), serum 8–20 mg/dL [2.9–7.1 mmol/L] Marbled $	Urea, an end product of protein metabolism, is excreted by the kidney. BUN is directly related to protein intake and nitrogen metabolism and inversely related to the rate of excretion of urea. Urea concentration in glomerular filtrate is the same as in plasma, but its tubular reabsorption is inversely related to the rate of urine formation. Thus, the BUN is a less useful measure of glomerular filtration rate than the serum creatinine (Cr).	**Increased in:** Renal failure (acute or chronic), urinary tract obstruction, dehydration, shock, burns, CHF, GI bleeding. Nephrotoxic drugs (eg, gentamicin). **Decreased in:** Hepatic failure, nephrotic syndrome, cachexia (low-protein and high-carbohydrate diets).	Urease assay method commonly used. BUN/Cr ratio (normally 12:1–20:1) is decreased in acute tubular necrosis, advanced liver disease, low protein intake, and following hemodialysis. BUN/Cr ratio is increased in dehydration, GI bleeding, and increased catabolism. Ref: N Engl J Med 1971;285:385.
***Brucella* serology**, serum < 1:80 titer Marbled $	Patients with acute brucellosis generally develop an agglutinating antibody titer of ≥ 1:160 within 3 weeks. The titer may rise during the acute infection, with relapses, brucellergen skin testing, or use of certain vaccines (see Interpretation). The agglutinin titer usually declines after 3 months or after successful therapy. Low titers may persist for years.	**Increased in:** *Brucella* infection (other than *B canis*) (97% within 3 weeks of illness); recent Brucellergen skin test; infections with *Francisella tularensis*, *Yersinia enterocolitica*, *Salmonella*, Rocky mountain spotted fever; vaccinations for cholera and tularemia. **Normal in:** *Brucella canis* infection.	This test will detect antibodies against all of the *Brucella* species except *B canis*. A fourfold or greater rise in titer in separate specimens drawn 1–4 weeks apart is indicative of recent exposure. Final diagnosis depends on isolation of organism by culture. Ref: J Infect Dis 1989;159:219. Ref: J Clin Microbiol 1980;11:691.

Test/Range/Collection	Physiologic Basis	Interpretation (sensitivity)	Comments
C-peptide, serum 0.8–4.0 ng/mL [µg/L] Marbled $$$ Fasting sample preferred.	C-peptide is an inactive by-product of the cleavage of proinsulin to active insulin. Its presence indicates endogenous release of insulin. C-peptide is largely excreted by the kidney.	**Increased in:** Renal failure, ingestion of oral hypoglycemic drugs, insulinomas, B cell transplants. **Decreased in:** Factitious hypoglycemia due to insulin administration, pancreatectomy, type I diabetes (decreased or undetectable).	Test is most useful to detect factitious insulin injection (increased insulin, decreased C-peptide) or to detect endogenous insulin production in diabetic patients receiving insulin (C-peptide present). Ref: Am J Med 1989;86:335. Ref: Arch Intern Med 1977;137:625.
Calcitonin, plasma Male: < 90 Female: < 70 pg/mL [ng/L] Green $$$ Fasting sample required. Place on ice.	Calcitonin is a 32-amino-acid polypeptide hormone secreted by the parafollicular C cells of the thyroid. It decreases osteoclastic bone resorption and lowers serum calcium levels.	**Increased in:** Medullary thyroid carcinoma (> 500 pg/mL on 2 occasions), Zollinger-Ellison syndrome, pernicious anemia, pregnancy (at term), newborns, carcinoma (breast, lung, pancreas), chronic renal failure.	Test is useful to diagnose and monitor medullary thyroid carcinoma, although stimulation tests may be necessary (eg, pentagastrin test [0.5 mg/kg over 10–150 seconds]; positive response is a 1.5-minute calcitonin level of > 190 pg/mL [male] or > 80 pg/mL [female]). Ref: Mayo Clin Proc 1975;50:53.

Calcium, serum		
Calcium, serum (Ca^{2+}) 8.5–10.5 mg/dL [2.1–2.6 mmol/L] ***Panic:*** < 6.5 or > 13.5 mg/dL Marbled $ Prolonged venous stasis during collection causes false increase in serum calcium.	Serum calcium is the sum of ionized calcium plus complexed calcium and calcium bound to proteins (mostly albumin). Level of ionized calcium is regulated by parathyroid hormone and vitamin D.	**Increased in:** Hyperparathyroidism, malignancies secreting PTH-like substances (especially squamous cell carcinoma of lung and renal cell carcinoma), vitamin D excess, milk-alkali syndrome, multiple myeloma, Paget's disease of bone with immobilization, sarcoidosis, other granulomatous disorders, familial hypocalciuria, vitamin A intoxication, thyrotoxicosis, Addison's disease. Drugs: antacids (some), calcium salts, chronic diuretic use (eg, thiazides), lithium, others. **Decreased in:** Hypoparathyroidism, vitamin D deficiency, renal insufficiency, pseudohypoparathyroidism, magnesium deficiency, hyperphosphatemia, massive transfusion, hypoalbuminemia.	Need to know serum albumin to interpret calcium level. For every decrease in albumin by 1 mg/dL, calcium should be corrected upward by 0.8 mg/dL. Ref: Ann Intern Med 1990;112:499.

	Calcium, urine	
Test/Range/Collection	**Physiologic Basis**	**Interpretation (sensitivity)**	**Comments**

Test/Range/Collection	Physiologic Basis	Interpretation (sensitivity)	Comments
Calcium, urine (U_{Ca}) 100–300 mg/d [2.5–7.5 mmol/d] Urine bottle containing hydrochloric acid $$$ Collect 24-hour urine.	Ordinarily there is moderate urinary calcium excretion, the amount depending on dietary calcium, parathyroid hormone (PTH) level, and protein intake.	**Increased in:** Hyperparathyroidism, osteolytic bone metastases, myeloma, osteoporosis, vitamin D intoxication, distal RTA, idiopathic hypercalciuria, thyrotoxicosis, Paget's disease, Fanconi's syndrome, hepatolenticular degeneration, schistosomiasis, sarcoidosis, malignancy (breast, bladder), osteitis deformans, immobilization. Drugs: acetazolamide, calcium salts, cholestyramine, corticosteroids, dihydrotachysterol, initial diuretic use (eg, furosemide), others. **Decreased in:** Hypoparathyroidism, pseudohypoparathyroidism, rickets, osteomalacia, nephrotic syndrome, acute glomerulonephritis, osteoblastic bone metastases, hypothyroidism, celiac disease, steatorrhea, hypocalciuric hypercalcemia, other causes of hypocalcemia. Drugs: bicarbonate, chronic diuretic use (eg, thiazides, chlorthalidone), estrogens, lithium, neomycin, oral contraceptives.	Approximately one-third of patients with hyperparathyroidism have normal urine calcium excretion. The extent of calcium excretion can be expressed as a urine calcium (U_{Ca})/ urine creatinine (U_{Cr}) ratio. Normally, $$\frac{U_{Ca}\ (mg/dL)}{U_{Cr}\ (mg/dL)} < 0.14$$ $$\frac{U_{Ca}\ (mmol/L)}{U_{Cr}\ (mmol/L)} < 0.40$$ Hypercalciuria is defined as a ratio > 0.20 or > 0.57, respectively. Test is useful in the evaluation of patients with renal stones. It is not usually needed for the diagnosis of hyperparathyroidism, which can be made using serum calcium (see above) and PTH measurements (see p 112). It may be useful in hypercalcemic patients to rule out familial hypocalciuric hypercalcemia. Ref: Ann Rev Med 1981;32:457.

	Carbon dioxide	Carboxyhemoglobin
Carbon dioxide (CO_2), total, serum (bicarbonate) 22–28 meq/L [mmol/L] *Panic:* < 15 or > 40 meq/L [mmol/L] Marbled $ Do not leave exposed to air since this will cause falsely low CO_2 levels.	Bicarbonate-carbonic acid buffer is one of the most important buffer systems in maintaining normal body fluid pH. Total CO_2 is measured as the sum of bicarbonate concentration plus carbonic acid concentration plus dissolved CO_2. Since bicarbonate makes up 90–95% of the total CO_2 content, total CO_2 is a useful surrogate for bicarbonate concentration.	**Increased in:** Primary metabolic alkalosis, compensated respiratory acidosis, volume contraction, mineralocorticoid excess, congenital chloridorrhea. Drugs: diuretics (eg, thiazide, furosemide). **Decreased in:** Metabolic acidosis, compensated respiratory alkalosis. Fanconi's syndrome, volume overload. Drugs: acetazolamide, outdated tetracycline.	Total CO_2 determination is indicated for all seriously ill patients on admission. If arterial blood gas studies are done, total CO_2 test is redundant. Simultaneous measurement of pH and PCO_2 is required to fully characterize a patient's acid-base status.
Carboxyhemoglobin, whole blood (HbCO) < 9% [< 0.09] Lavender $$ Do not remove stopper.	Carbon monoxide (CO) combines irreversibly with hemoglobin at the sites that normally bind oxygen. This produces a decrease in oxygen saturation and a shift in the oxyhemoglobin dissociation curve, resulting in decreased release of oxygen to the tissues.	**Increased in:** Carbon monoxide poisoning. Exposure to automobile exhaust or smoke from fires. Cigarette smokers can have up to 9% carboxyhemoglobin, nonsmokers have < 2%.	Test (if available within minutes, together with O_2 saturation by oximeter) is useful in evaluation of CO poisoning. PO_2 is usually normal in CO poisoning. Test measures carboxyhemoglobin spectrophotometrically. Ref: N Engl J Med 1989;321:1474.

Test/Range/Collection	Physiologic Basis	Interpretation (sensitivity)	Comments
Carcinoembryonic antigen (CEA)		**Carcinoembryonic antigen**	
Carcinoembryonic antigen, serum (CEA) 0–2.5 ng/mL [µg/L] Marbled $$	CEA is an oncofetal antigen, a glycoprotein associated with certain malignancies, particularly epithelial tumors.	**Increased in:** Colon cancer (72%), lung cancer (76%), pancreatic cancer (91%), stomach cancer (61%), cigarette smokers, benign liver disease (acute 50% and chronic 90%), benign GI disease (peptic ulcer, pancreatitis, colitis). Elevations > 20 ng/mL are generally associated with malignancy.	Screening: Test is not sensitive or specific enough to be useful in cancer screening. Monitoring after surgery: Test is used to follow progression of colon cancer after surgery (elevated CEA levels suggest recurrence 3–6 months before other clinical indicators), although such monitoring has not yet been shown to improve survival rates. If monitoring is done, the same assay method must be consistently used in order to eliminate any method-dependent variability. Ref: Ann Intern Med 1986;104:66. Ref: Ann Intern Med 1981;94:407.

CD4/CD8 ratio	Ceruloplasmin
CD4/CD8 ratio, whole blood Ratio: 0.8–2.9 CD4: 359–1725 cells/μL (29–61%) CD8: 177–1106 cells/μL (18–42%) Lavender $$$ If an absolute CD4 count is required, also request a CBC and differential.	**Ceruloplasmin, serum** 20–35 mg/dL [200–350 mg/L] Marbled $$
Lymphocyte identification depends on specific cell surface antigens (clusters of differentiation, CD), which can be detected with monoclonal antibodies using flow cytometry. CD4 cells are predominantly helper-inducer cells of the immunologic system. They react with peptide class II major histocompatibility complex antigens and augment B cell responses and T cell lymphokine secretion. CD8 cells can be divided into suppressor cells, which decrease B cell responses, and cytotoxic T cells.	Ceruloplasmin, a 120,000-160,000 MW α_2 glycoprotein synthesized by the liver, is the main (95%) copper-carrying protein in human serum.
Increased in: Rheumatoid arthritis, type I diabetes mellitus, SLE without renal disease, primary biliary cirrhosis, atopic dermatitis, Sézary syndrome, psoriasis, chronic autoimmune hepatitis. **Decreased in:** AIDS/HIV infection, SLE with renal disease, acute CMV infection, burns, graft-versus-host disease, sunburn, myelodysplasia syndromes, acute lymphocytic leukemia in remission, recovery from bone marrow transplantation, herpes infection, infectious mononucleosis, measles, ataxia-telangiectasia, vigorous exercise.	**Increased in:** Acute and chronic inflammation, pregnancy. Drugs: oral contraceptives, phenytoin. **Decreased in:** Wilson's disease (hepatolenticular degeneration) (95%), CNS disease other than Wilson's (15%), liver disease other than Wilson's (23%), malabsorption, malnutrition, primary biliary cirrhosis, nephrotic syndrome, severe copper deficiency, Menkes' disease (X-linked inherited copper deficiency).
Progressive decline in the number and function of CD4 lymphocytes seems to be the most characteristic immunologic defect in AIDS. Absolute CD4 measurement is particularly useful (more useful than the CD4/CD8 ratio) in determining eligibility for therapy and in monitoring the progress of the disease. Absolute CD4 count depends, analytically, on the reliability of the white blood cell differential count, as well as on the percentage of CD4 cells identified using the appropriate monoclonal antibody. Ref: Hem Onc Clin N Am 1991; 5(2):215. Ref: Semin Immunol 1990;2(6):419.	Slitlamp examination for Kayser-Fleischer rings and serum ceruloplasmin level recommended for diagnosis of Wilson's disease. Serum copper level is very rarely indicated. 5% of patients with Wilson's disease have low-normal levels of ceruloplasmin. Ref: Q J Med 1979;48:447. Ref: Q J Med 1987;65:959.

Test/Range/Collection	Physiologic Basis	Interpretation (sensitivity)	Comments
Chloride, serum (Cl⁻) 98–107 meq/L [mmol/L] Marbled $	Chloride, the principal inorganic anion of extracellular fluid, is important in maintaining normal acid-base balance and normal osmolality. If chloride is lost (as HCl or NH_4Cl), alkalosis ensues; if chloride is ingested or retained, acidosis ensues.	**Increased in:** Renal failure, nephrotic syndrome, renal tubular acidosis, dehydration, overtreatment with saline, hyperparathyroidism, diabetes insipidus, metabolic acidosis from diarrhea (loss of HCO_3^-), respiratory alkalosis, hyperadrenocorticism. Drugs: acetazolamide (hyperchloremic acidosis), androgens, hydrochlorothiazide, salicylates (intoxication). **Decreased in:** Vomiting, diarrhea, gastrointestinal suction, renal failure combined with salt deprivation, overtreatment with diuretics, chronic respiratory acidosis, diabetic ketoacidosis, excessive sweating, SIADH, salt-losing nephropathy, acute intermittent porphyria, water intoxication, expansion of extracellular fluid volume, adrenal insufficiency, hyperaldosteronism, metabolic alkalosis. Drugs: chronic laxative or bicarbonate ingestion, corticosteroids, diuretics.	

Chloride

	Cholesterol	
Cholesterol, serum Desirable < 200 Borderline 200–239 High risk > 240 mg/dL [Desirable < 5.2 Borderline 5.2–6.1 High risk > 6.2 mmol/L] Marbled $ Fasting preferred.	Cholesterol level is determined by lipid metabolism, which is in turn influenced by heredity, diet, and other liver, kidney, thyroid, and endocrine organ functions. Total cholesterol (TC) = low density lipoprotein (LDL) cholesterol + high density lipoprotein (HDL) cholesterol + (triglycerides [TG]/5) (valid only if TG < 400). Since LDL cholesterol is the clinically important entity, it is calculated as $LDL = TC - HDL - (TG/5)$. This calculation is valid only if specimen is obtained fasting (in order to obtain relevant triglyceride and HDL levels).	**Increased in:** *Primary disorders:* polygenic hypercholesterolemia. familial hypercholesterolemia (deficiency of LDL receptor), familial combined hyperlipidemia, familial dysbetalipoproteinemia. *Secondary disorders:* hypothyroidism, uncontrolled diabetes mellitus, nephrotic syndrome, biliary obstruction, anorexia nervosa, hepatoma, Cushing's syndrome, acute intermittent porphyria. Drugs: corticosteroids. **Decreased in:** Severe liver disease (acute hepatitis, cirrhosis, malignancy), hyperthyroidism, severe acute or chronic illness, malnutrition, extensive burns, Gaucher's disease, Tangier disease, abetalipoproteinemia, intestinal lymphangiectasia.	It is important to treat the cause of secondary hypercholesterolemia (eg, hypothyroidism). National Cholesterol Education Program Expert Panel has published clinical recommendations for cholesterol management (see first reference). Ref: Arch Intern Med 1988;148:36. Ref: Ann Intern Med 1989;110:622.

	Chorionic gonadotropin		
Test/Range/Collection	Physiologic Basis	Interpretation (sensitivity)	Comments
Chorionic gonado-tropin, ß-subunit, quantitative, serum (ß-hCG) Males and nonpreg-nant females: undetectable or < 2 mIU/mL [IU/L] Marbled $$	Human chorionic gonadotropin is a glycoprotein made up of 2 sub-units (α and β). Human glycopro-teins such as LH, FSH, and TSH share the α subunit of hCG, but the β subunit is specific for hCG. hCG is produced by trophoblastic tissue, and its detection in serum or urine is the basis for pregnancy testing. Serum hCG can be detected as early as 24 hours after implantation at a concentration of 5 mIU/mL. During normal pregnancy, serum levels double every 2–3 days and are 50–100 mIU/mL at the time of the first missed menstrual period. Peak levels are reached 60–80 days after the last menstrual period (LMP) (30,000–100,000 mIU/mL), and levels then decrease to a plateau of 5,000–10,000 mIU/mL at about 120 days after LMP and persist until delivery.	**Increased in:** Pregnancy, trophoblas-tic tumors (hydatidiform mole, choriocarcinoma of uterus), some germ cell tumors (teratomas of ovary or testicle, seminoma), ectopic hCG production by other malignancies (stomach, pancreas, lung, colon, liver). Failure of elevated serum lev-els to decrease after surgical resec-tion of trophoblastic tumor indicates metastatic tumor; levels rising from normal indicate tumor recurrence. **Decreasing over time:** Threatened abortion.	Routine pregnancy testing is done by *qualitative* serum or urine hCG test. Test will be positive (> 50 mIU/mL) in most pregnant women at the time of or shortly after the first missed menstrual period. *Quantitative* hCG testing is indicated for (1) the evaluation of suspected ectopic pregnancy (where levels are lower than in normal pregnancy at the same gesta-tional age) if the routine pregnancy test is negative; (2) the evaluation of threat-ened abortion. In both situations, hCG levels fail to demonstrate the normal early pregnancy increase. Test is also indicated for following the course of trophoblastic tumors. Ref: J Clin Endocrinol Metab 1988; 66:538. Ref: Am J Obstet Gynecol 1977; 127:711. Ref: Ann Emerg Med 1985;14:1074.

	C difficile enterotoxin	Clotting time
Clostridium difficile enterotoxin, stool Negative ($\leq$ 1:10 titer) Urine or stool container $$$ Must be tested within 12 hours of collection as toxin (B) is labile.	*Clostridium difficile*, a motile, gram-positive rod, is the major recognized agent of antibiotic-associated diarrhea, which is toxigenic in origin (see Antibiotic-associated colitis, p 174). There are 2 toxins (A and B) produced by *C difficile*. Cell culture is used to detect the cytopathic effect of the toxins, whose identity is confirmed by neutralization with specific antitoxins. Toxin A (more weakly cytopathic in cell culture) is enterotoxic and reproduces enteric disease. Toxin B (more easily detected in standard cell culture assays) fails to produce intestinal disease.	**Positive in:** Antibiotic-associated diarrhea (15–25%), antibiotic-associated colitis (50–75%), and pseudomembranous colitis (90–100%). About 3% of healthy adults and 10–20% of hospitalized patients have *C difficile* in their colonic flora. There is also a high carrier rate of *C difficile* and its toxin in healthy neonates.	Definitive diagnosis of disease caused by *C difficile* toxin is by endoscopic detection of pseudomembranous colitis. Direct examination of stool for leukocytes, gram-positive rods, or blood is not helpful. Culture of *C difficile* is not routinely performed, as it would isolate numerous nontoxigenic *C difficile* strains. Ref: Rev Infect Dis 1990;12:S243. Ref: CRC Crit Rev Clin Lab Sci 1986; 24:235.
Clotting time, activated, whole blood (ACT) 114–186 seconds Special black tube $$ Performed at patient bedside. Avoid traumatic venipuncture, which may cause contamination with tissue juices and decrease clotting time.	A bedside or operating room test that assesses heparinization by measuring time taken for whole blood to clot.	**Prolonged in:** Heparin therapy, severe deficiency of clotting factors (except factors VII and XIII), functional platelet disorders, afibrinogenemia, circulating anticoagulants. **Normal in:** Thrombocytopenia, factor VII deficiency, von Willebrand's disease.	Many consider this test unreliable. Reproducibility of prolonged ACTs is poor. Used only to document intraoperative or dialysis-related heparin neutralization. Should not be used to regulate therapeutic heparin dosage adjustments; use partial thromboplastin time (PTT) instead. Ref: Ann Thorac Surg 1978;26:231.

	Coccidioides serology		Cold agglutinins
Test/Range/Collection	Physiologic Basis	Interpretation (sensitivity)	Comments
Coccidioides serology, serum or CSF Negative Marbled $$	Screens for presence of antibodies to *Coccidioides immitis*. IgM antibodies appear early in disease in 80% of patients, begin to decrease after the third week, and are rarely seen after 5 months. They may persist in disseminated cases. IgG antibodies appear later in the course of the disease.	**Positive in:** Infection by *Coccidioides* (90%). **Negative in:** Coccidioidin skin testing, many patients with chronic cavitary *Coccidioides*; 5% of meningeal *Coccidioides* is negative by CSF complement fixation (CF) test.	Precipitin and CF tests detect 90% of primary symptomatic cases. Precipitin test is most effective in detecting early primary infection or an exacerbation of existing disease. Test is diagnostic but not prognostic. CF test becomes positive later than precipitin test, and titers can be used to assess severity of infection. Titers rise as the disease progresses and decline as the patient improves. Ref: Rose NR et al (editors): *Manual of Clinical Laboratory Immunology.* American Society for Microbiology, 1986.
Cold agglutinins, plasma < 1:20 titer Lavender or blue $$ Specimen should be kept at 37 °C.	Detects antibodies that agglutinate red blood cells in the cold (strongly at 4 °C, weakly at 24 °C, and weakly or not at all at 37 °C). These antibodies are present in primary atypical pneumonias due to *Mycoplasma pneumoniae*, in certain autoimmune hemolytic anemias, and in normal persons (not clinically significant).	**Increased in:** Chronic cold agglutinin disease, lymphoproliferative disorders (eg, Waldenström's macroglobulinemia), autoimmune hemolytic anemia, collagen-vascular diseases, *M pneumoniae* pneumonia, infectious mononucleosis, mumps orchitis, cytomegalovirus, tropical diseases (eg, trypanosomiasis).	In *Mycoplasma* pneumonia, titers rise early, are maximal at 3–4 weeks after onset, and then disappear rapidly. These antibodies are usually IgM anti-I antibodies distinct from antibodies to *M pneumoniae*. A rise in cold agglutinin antibody titer is suggestive of recent *Mycoplasma* infection but is found in other diseases. Ref: N Engl J Med 1977;297:583.

	Complement C3	Complement C4
Complement C3, serum 64–166 mg/dL [640–1660 mg/L] Marbled $$	The classic and alternative complement pathways converge at the C3 step in the complement cascade. Low levels indicate activation by one or both pathways. Most diseases with immune complexes will show decreased C3 levels. Test is usually performed as an immunoassay (by radial immunodiffusion or nephelometry).	**Increased in:** Many inflammatory conditions as an acute phase reactant, active phase of rheumatic diseases (eg, rheumatoid arthritis, SLE), acute viral hepatitis, myocardial infarction, cancer, diabetes, pregnancy, sarcoidosis, amyloidosis, thyroiditis. **Decreased by:** Decreased synthesis (protein malnutrition, congenital deficiency, severe liver disease), increased catabolism (immune complex disease, membranoproliferative glomerulonephritis [75%], SLE, Sjögren's syndrome, rheumatoid arthritis, disseminated intravascular coagulation, paroxysmal nocturnal hemoglobinuria, autoimmune hemolytic anemia, gram-negative bacteremia), increased loss (burns, gastroenteropathies).	Complement C3 levels may be useful in following the activity of immune complex diseases. The best test to detect inherited deficiencies is CH_{50}. Ref: N Engl J Med 1987;316:1525.
Complement C4, serum 15–45 mg/dL [150–450 mg/L] Marbled $$	C4 is a component of the classic complement pathway. Depressed levels usually indicate classic pathway activation.	**Increased in:** Various malignancies (not clinically useful). **Decreased by:** Decreased synthesis (congenital deficiency), increased catabolism (SLE, rheumatoid arthritis, proliferative glomerulonephritis, hereditary angioedema), and increased loss (burns, protein-losing enteropathies).	Low C4 accompanies acute attacks of hereditary angioedema, and C4 is used as a first-line test for the disease. C1 esterase inhibitor levels are not indicated for the evaluation of hereditary angioedema unless C4 is low. Congenital C4 deficiency occurs with an SLE-like syndrome. Test is usually performed as an immunoassay and not a functional assay. Ref: N Engl J Med 1987;316:1525.

Test/Range/Collection	Physiologic Basis	Interpretation (sensitivity)	Comments
Complement CH$_{50}$, plasma or serum (CH$_{50}$) 22–40 U/mL (laboratory-specific) Marbled $$$	The quantitative assay of hemolytic complement activity depends on the ability of the classic complement pathway to induce hemolysis of red cells sensitized with optimal amounts of anti-red cell antibodies. For precise titrations of hemolytic complement, the dilution of serum that will lyse 50% of the indicator red cells is determined as the CH$_{50}$. This arbitrary unit depends on the conditions of the assay and is therefore laboratory-specific.	**Decreased with:** > 50–80% deficiency of classic pathway complement components (congenital or acquired deficiencies). **Normal in:** Deficiencies of the alternative pathway complement components.	This is a functional assay of biologic activity. Sensitivity to decreased levels of complement components depends on exactly how the test is performed. It is used to detect congenital and acquired severe deficiency disorders of the classic complement pathway. Ref: N Engl J Med 1987;316:1525.
Cortisol, plasma or serum 8:00 AM: 5–20 µg/dL [140–550 nmol/L] Marbled, lavender, or green $$	Release of corticotropin-releasing factor (CRF) from the hypothalamus stimulates release of ACTH from the pituitary, which in turn stimulates release of cortisol from the adrenal. Cortisol provides negative feedback to this system. Test measures both free cortisol and cortisol bound to cortisol-binding globulin (CBG). Morning levels are higher than evening levels.	**Increased in:** Cushing's syndrome, acute illness, surgery, trauma, depression, anxiety, alcoholism, starvation, chronic renal failure, increased CBG (congenital, pregnancy, estrogen therapy). **Decreased in:** Addison's disease; decreased CBG (congenital, liver disease, nephrotic syndrome).	Cortisol levels are useful only in the context of standardized suppression or stimulation tests. (See Cosyntropin stimulation test, p 69, and Dexamethasone suppression tests, p 73). Circadian fluctuations in cortisol levels limit usefulness of single measurements. Analysis of diurnal variation of cortisol is not useful diagnostically. Ref: Metabolism 1979;28:955.

Cortisol (urinary-free)	Cosyntropin stimulation test
This test replaces both the assessment of 17-hydroxycorticosteroids and the 17-ketogenic steroids in the initial diagnosis of Cushing's syndrome. Not useful for the diagnosis of adrenal insufficiency. Ref: Metabolism 1979;28:955.	Test does not distinguish primary from secondary (pituitary) adrenal insufficiency, since in secondary adrenal insufficiency the atrophic adrenal may be unresponsive to cosyntropin. Test may not reliably detect pituitary insufficiency. Metyrapone test may be useful to assess the pituitary-adrenal axis (see Metyrapone test, p 107). Ref: Lancet 1965;1:243.
Increased in: Cushing's syndrome, acute illness, stress. **Not increased in:** Obesity.	**Decreased in:** Adrenal insufficiency, pituitary insufficiency.
Urinary-free cortisol measurement is useful in the initial evaluation of suspected Cushing's syndrome (see Cushing's syndrome algorithm, p 252).	Cosyntropin (synthetic ACTH preparation) stimulates the adrenal to release cortisol. A normal response is a doubling of basal levels or an increment of 7 μg/dL (200nmol/L) to a level above 18 μg/dL (> 504 nmol/L). A poor cortisol response to cosyntropin indicates adrenal insufficiency (see Adrenocortical insufficiency algorithm, p 250).
Cortisol (urinary-free), urine 10–110 μg/24 h [30–300 nmol/d] Urine bottle containing boric acid. $$$ Collect 24-hour urine.	**Cosyntropin stimulation test,** serum or plasma Marbled, green, or lavender $$$ First draw a cortisol level. Then administer cosyntropin (0.25 mg IV). Draw another cortisol level in 30 minutes.

Test/Range/Collection	Physiologic Basis	Interpretation (sensitivity)	Comments
Creatine kinase, serum (CK) 32–267 IU/L [0.53–4.45 µkat/L] (method-dependent) Marbled $	Creatine kinase splits creatine phosphate in the presence of ADP to yield creatine and ATP. Skeletal muscle, myocardium, and brain are rich in the enzyme. CK is released by tissue damage.	**Increased in:** Myocardial infarction, myocarditis, muscle trauma, rhabdomyolysis, muscular dystrophy, polymyositis, severe muscular exertion, malignant hyperthermia, hypothyroidism, cerebral infarction, Reye's syndrome, tetanus, surgery, generalized convulsions, alcoholism, IM injections, DC countershock. Drugs: clofibrate.	CK is as sensitive a test as aldolase for muscle damage, so aldolase is not needed. During a myocardial infarction, serum CK level rises rapidly (within 3–5 hours); elevation persists for 2–3 days post-myocardial infarction. In the CCU, increased CK has a sensitivity of 97% and specificity of 67% for diagnosis of myocardial infarction. Ref: Arch Intern Med 1987;147:115. Ref: Ann Intern Med 1986;105:221.
Creatine kinase MB, serum (CKMB) < 16 IU/L [< 0.27 µkat/L] or < 4% of total CK (laboratory-specific) Marbled $$	CK consists of 3 isoenzymes, made up of 2 subunits, M and B. The fraction with the greatest electrophoretic mobility is CK1 (BB); CK2 (MB) is intermediate and CK3 (MM) moves slowest. Skeletal muscle is characterized by isoenzyme MM and brain by isoenzyme BB. Myocardium has approximately 40% MB isoenzyme. Assay techniques include isoenzyme separation by electrophoresis or immunoassay using antibody specific for MB fraction.	**Increased in:** Myocardial infarction, cardiac trauma, certain muscular dystrophies, and polymyositis. Slight persistent elevation reported in a few patients on hemodialysis.	Test result may be reported either as CKMB "present" or "absent," or there may be quantitation of isoenzyme. Laboratory-specific reference ranges must be used. CKMB is a relatively specific test for myocardial infarction. It appears in serum approximately 4 hours after infarction, peaks at 12–24 hours, and declines over 48–72 hours. CKMB should not be ordered as a screening test because a single normal CKMB does not rule out myocardial infarction. Estimation of CKMM and CKBB is not clinically useful. Use total CK. Ref: Clin Chem 1989;35:7. Ref: Clin Biochem 1988;21:211.

	Creatinine	Creatinine clearance
Creatinine, serum (Cr) 0.6–1.2 mg/dL [50–100 µmol/L] Marbled $	Endogenous creatinine is excreted by filtration through the glomerulus and by tubular secretion. Creatinine clearance is an acceptable clinical measure of glomerular filtration rate (GFR), though it sometimes overestimates GFR. For each 50% reduction in GFR, serum creatinine approximately doubles.	**Increased in:** Acute or chronic renal failure, urinary tract obstruction, nephrotoxic drugs. **Decreased in:** Reduced muscle mass.	In alkaline picrate method, substances other than Cr (eg, acetoacetate, acetone, β-hydroxybutyrate, α-ketoglutarate, pyruvate, glucose) may give falsely high results. Therefore, patients with diabetic ketoacidosis may have spuriously elevated Cr. Cephalosporins may spuriously increase or decrease Cr measurement. Increased bilirubin may spuriously decrease Cr. Ref: Clin Chem 1990;36:1951.
Creatinine clearance, (Cl$_{Cr}$) Adults: 90–130 mL/min/1.73 m^2 BSA $$ Collect carefully-timed 24-hour urine and simultaneous serum/plasma creatinine sample. Record patient's weight and height.	Widely used test of glomerular filtration rate (GFR). Theoretically reliable, but often compromised by incomplete urine collection. Creatinine clearance is calculated from measurement of urine creatinine (U$_{Cr}$ [mg/dL]), plasma/serum creatinine (P$_{Cr}$ [mg/dL]), and urine flow rate ($\dot{V}$ [mL/min]) according to the formula:$$Cl_{Cr}(mL/min) = \frac{U_{Cr} \times V}{P_{Cr}}$$Creatinine clearance is often "corrected" for body surface area (BSA [m^2]) according to the formula:$$Cl_{Cr}\text{(corrected)} = Cl_{Cr}\text{(uncorrected)} \times \frac{1.73}{BSA}$$	**Increased in:** High cardiac output, exercise, acromegaly, diabetes mellitus (early stage), infections, hypothyroidism. **Decreased in:** Acute or chronic renal failure, decreased renal blood flow (shock, hemorrhage, dehydration, CHF). Drugs: nephrotoxic drugs.	Serum Cr may, in practice, be a more reliable indicator of renal function than Cl$_{Cr}$ unless urine collection is carefully monitored. Cl$_{Cr}$ will overestimate GFR to the extent that Cr is secreted by the renal tubules. Cl$_{Cr}$ can be estimated from the serum creatinine using the following formula:$$\frac{Cl_{Cr}}{(mL/min)} = \frac{(140 - age) \times Wt\ (kg)}{72 \times P_{Cr}}$$Ref: N Engl J Med 1962;266:317. Ref: Acta Med Scand 1974;196:517.

Test/Range/Collection	Physiologic Basis	Interpretation (sensitivity)	Comments
Cryoglobulins, serum < 0.12 mg/mL Marbled $ Must be immediately transported to lab at 37 °C.	Cryoglobulins are immunoglobulins (IgG, IgM, IgA, or light chains) which precipitate on exposure to the cold. Type I cryoglobulins (25%) are monoclonal proteins, most commonly IgM, occasionally IgG, and rarely IgA or Bence Jones protein, seen in multiple myeloma and Waldenström's macroglobulinemia. Type II (25%) are mixed cryoglobulins with a monoclonal component (usually IgM but occasionally IgG or IgA) that complexes with autologous normal IgG in the cryoprecipitate. Type III (50%) are mixed polyclonal cryoglobulins (IgM and IgG).	**Increased in:** Immunoproliferative disorders (multiple myeloma, Waldenström's macroglobulinemia, chronic lymphocytic leukemia, lymphoma), collagen-vascular disease (SLE, polyarteritis nodosa, rheumatoid arthritis), hemolytic anemia, essential mixed cryoglobulinemia, hepatitis B infection.	All types of cryoglobulins may cause cold-induced symptoms including Raynaud's phenomenon, vascular purpura, and urticaria. Patients with type II and III cryoglobulinemia often have immune complex disease, with vascular purpura, arthritis, and nephritis. Typing of cryoglobulins by electrophoresis is not necessary for diagnosis or clinical management. Ref: JAMA 1982;248:2670 Ref: Am J Med 1980;68:757.
Cytomegalovirus (CMV) antibody, serum Negative Marbled $$$	Detects the presence of antibody to CMV, either IgG or IgM. CMV infection is usually acquired during childhood or early adulthood. By age 20–40 years, 40–90% of the population has CMV antibodies.	**Increased in:** Previous or active CMV infection. False-positive CMV IgM tests occur when rheumatoid factor or infectious mononucleosis is present.	Serial specimens exhibiting a > 4-fold titer rise suggest a recent infection. Active CMV infection must be documented by viral isolation. Useful for screening of potential organ donors and recipients. Detection of CMV IgM antibody in the serum of a newborn usually indicates congenital infection. Detection of CMV IgG antibody is not diagnostic, since maternal CMV IgG antibody passed via the placenta can persist in newborn's serum for 6 months. Ref: Rev Infect Dis 1988;10:S468.

Dexamethasone suppression tests		
Dexamethasone suppression test (single low-dose, overnight), serum 8:00 AM serum cortisol level: < 5 µg/dL [< 140 nmol/L] $ Give 1 mg dexamethasone at 11:00 PM. At 8:00 AM draw serum cortisol level.	In normal patients, dexamethasone suppresses the 8:00 AM serum cortisol level to below 5 µg/dL. Patients with Cushing's syndrome have 8:00 AM levels > 10 µg/dL (> 276 nmol/L).	**Positive in:** Cushing's syndrome (98%, 98% specificity in lean outpatients), obese patients (13%), hospitalized or chronically ill patients (23%).	Good screening test for Cushing's syndrome. If this test is abnormal, use high-dose test (see below) to determine etiology. (See also Cushing's syndrome algorithm, p 252.) Patients taking phenytoin may fail to suppress because of enhanced dexamethasone metabolism. Depressed patients may also fail to suppress morning cortisol level. Ref: Metabolism 1979;28:955.
Dexamethasone suppression test (high-dose, overnight), serum 8:00 AM serum cortisol level: < 5 µg/dL [< 140 nmol/L] $ Give 8 mg dexamethasone dose at 11:00 PM. At 8:00 AM draw cortisol level.	Suppression of plasma cortisol levels to < 50% of baseline with dexamethasone indicates Cushing's disease (pituitary-dependent ACTH hypersecretion) and differentiates this from adrenal and ectopic Cushing's syndrome (see Cushing's syndrome algorithm, p 252).	**Positive in:** Cushing's disease (92%, specificity 100%).	Test indicated only after a positive low-dose dexamethasone suppression test. Measurement of urinary 17-hydroxycorticosteroids has been replaced in this test by measurement of serum cortisol. Ref: Ann Intern Med 1986;104:180. Ref: Ann Intern Med 1990;112:434.

Test/Range/Collection	Physiologic Basis	Interpretation (sensitivity)	Comments
		Epstein-Barr virus antibodies	**Erythrocyte count**
Epstein-Barr virus antibodies, serum (EBV) Negative Marbled $$	Antiviral (IgM) capsid antibodies (anti-VCA) often reach their peak at clinical presentation and last up to 3 months; anti-VCA IgG antibodies last for life. Early antigen antibodies (anti-EA) are next to develop, are most often positive at 1 month after presentation, typically last for 2–3 months, and may last up to 6 months in low titers. Anti-EA may also be found in some patients with Hodgkin's disease, chronic lymphocytic leukemia, and some other malignancies. Anti-EB nuclear antigen (anti-EBNA) antibody begins to appear in a minority of patients in the third or fourth week but is uniformly present by 6 months.	**Increased in:** EB virus infection, infectious mononucleosis. Antibodies to the diffuse (D) form of antigen (detected in the cytoplasm and nucleus of infected cells) is greatly elevated in nasopharyngeal carcinoma. Antibodies to the restricted (R) form of antigen (detected only in the cytoplasm of infected cells) is greatly elevated in Burkitt's lymphoma.	Most useful in diagnosing infectious mononucleosis in patients who have the clinical and hematologic criteria for the disease but who fail to develop the heterophile agglutinins (10%) (see Heterophile agglutination, p 92). EBV antibodies cannot be used to diagnose "chronic" mononucleosis. Chronic fatigue syndrome is not caused by EBV. The best indicator of primary infection is a positive anti-VCA IgM (check for false-positives caused by rheumatoid factor). Ref: Rose NR et al (editors): *Manual of Clinical Laboratory Immunology.* American Society for Microbiology, 1986.
Erythrocyte count, whole blood (RBC count) $4.2\text{–}5.6 \times 10^6 /\mu L$ $[\times 10^{12}/L]$ Lavender $	Erythrocytes are counted by automated instruments using electrical impedance or light scattering.	**Increased in:** Secondary polycythemia (hemoconcentration), polycythemia vera. Spurious increase with increased white blood cells. **Decreased in:** Anemia. Spurious decrease with autoagglutination.	Ref: Lab Med 1983;14:509.

Test / Specimen	Physiologic basis	Interpretation	Comments
Erythrocyte sedimentation rate, whole blood (ESR) Male: < 10 Female: < 15 mm/h (laboratory-specific) Lavender $ Test must be run within 2 hours of sample collection.	In plasma, erythrocytes (red blood cells [RBCs]) usually settle slowly. However, if they aggregate for any reason (usually because of plasma proteins called acute phase reactants, eg, fibrinogen) they settle rapidly. Sedimentation of RBCs occurs because their density is greater than plasma. ESR measures the distance that erythrocytes fall in mm during 1 hour.	**Increased in:** Infections (osteomyelitis, pelvic inflammatory disease [75%]), inflammatory disease (temporal arteritis, polymyalgia rheumatica, rheumatic fever), malignant neoplasms, paraproteinemias, anemia, pregnancy, chronic renal failure, GI disease (ulcerative colitis, regional ileitis). **Decreased in:** Polycythemia, sickle cell anemia, spherocytosis, anisocytosis, hypofibrinogenemia, hypogammaglobulinemia, congestive heart failure, microcytosis. Drugs: high-dose corticosteroids.	There is a good correlation between ESR and C-reactive protein, but ESR is less expensive. Test is useful and indicated only for diagnosis and monitoring of temporal arteritis and polymyalgia rheumatica. The test is not sensitive or specific for other conditions. ESR is higher in women and older persons. Low value is of no diagnostic significance. Ref: Ann Intern Med 1986;104:515. Ref: Am J Med 1985;78:1001.
Erythropoietin, serum (EPO) 5–20 mIU/mL [4–26 IU/L] Marbled $$$	Erythropoietin is a glycoprotein hormone produced in the kidney that induces red blood cell production by stimulating proliferation, differentiation, and maturation of erythroid precursors. Hypoxia is the usual stimulus for production of EPO. In conditions of bone marrow hyporesponsiveness, EPO levels are elevated. In chronic renal failure, EPO production is decreased.	**Increased in:** Anemias associated with bone marrow hyporesponsiveness (aplastic anemia, iron deficiency anemia), secondary polycythemia (high-altitude hypoxia, COPD, pulmonary fibrosis), erythropoietin-producing tumors (cerebellar hemangioblastomas, pheochromocytomas, renal tumors), pregnancy, polycystic kidney disease. **Decreased in:** Anemia of chronic disease, renal failure, inflammatory states, primary polycythemia (polycythemia vera) (39%).	Test is not very useful in differentiating polycythemia vera from secondary polycythemia. Since virtually all patients with severe anemia due to chronic renal failure respond to EPO therapy, pretherapy EPO levels are not indicated. Ref: Transfusion 1989;29:46. Ref: N Engl J Med 1986;315:283.

Test/Range/Collection	Physiologic Basis	Interpretation (sensitivity)	Comments
Ethanol, serum (EtOH) 0 mg/dL [mmol/L] Marbled $$ Do not use alcohol swab. Do not remove stopper.	Measures serum level of ethyl alcohol (ethanol).	**Present in:** Ethanol ingestion.	Whole blood alcohol concentrations are about 15% lower than serum concentrations. Each 0.1 mg/dL of ethanol contributes about 22 mosm/kg to serum osmolality. Legal intoxication in many states is defined as > 0.08 mg/dL (> 17 mmol/L). Ref: N Engl J Med 1976;294:757.
Factor VIII assay, plasma 40–150% of normal, (varies with age) Blue $$$ Deliver immediately to laboratory on ice. Stable for 2 hours.	Measures activity of factor VIII (antihemophilic factor), a key factor of the intrinsic clotting cascade.	**Increased in:** Inflammatory states (acute phase reactant), last trimester of pregnancy, oral contraceptives. **Decreased in:** Hemophilia A, von Willebrand's disease, disseminated intravascular coagulation, acquired factor VIII antibodies.	Normal hemostasis requires at least 25% of factor VIII activity. Symptomatic hemophiliacs usually have levels ≤ 5%. Disease levels are defined as severe (< 1%), moderate (1–5%) and mild (>5%). Factor VIII assays are used to guide replacement therapy in patients with hemophilia. Ref: Semin Hematol 1967;4:93.

Fecal fat			
Fecal fat, stool Random: < 60 droplets of fat/ high power field 72 hour: < 7 g/day $$$ Qualitative: random stool sample is adequate. Quantitative: dietary fat should be at least 50–150 g/day for 2 days before collection. Then all stool should be collected for 72 hours and refrigerated.	In healthy people, most dietary fat is completely absorbed in the small intestine. Normal small intestinal lining, bile acids, and pancreatic enzymes are required for normal fat absorption.	**Increased in:** Malabsorption from small bowel disease (regional enteritis, celiac disease, tropical sprue), pancreatic insufficiency.	A random, qualitative fecal fat (so-called Sudan stain) is only useful if positive. Furthermore, it does not correlate well with quantitative measurements. Sudan stain appears to detect triglycerides and lipolytic by-products, whereas 72-hour fecal fat measures fatty acids from a variety of sources, including phospholipids, cholesteryl esters, and triglycerides. The quantitative method can be used to measure the degree of fat malabsorption initially and then after a therapeutic intervention. A normal quantitative stool fat reliably rules out pancreatic insufficiency and most forms of generalized small intestine disease. Ref: Gastroenterol Clin North Am 1989; 18:467.

Test/Range/Collection	Physiologic Basis	Interpretation (sensitivity)	Comments
Fecal occult blood, stool Negative $ Patient should be on a special diet free of exogenous peroxidase activity (meat, fish, turnips, horseradish), GI irritants (aspirin, non-steroidal anti-inflammatory drugs), and iron. To avoid false-negatives, patients should avoid taking vitamin C.	Measures blood in the stool using gum guaiac as an indicator reagent. In the Hemoccult test, gum guaiac is impregnated in a test paper that is smeared with stool using an applicator. Hydrogen peroxide is used as a developer solution. The resultant phenolic oxidation of guaiac in the presence of blood in the stool yields a blue color.	**Positive in:** Upper GI disease (peptic ulcer, gastritis, variceal bleeding, esophageal and gastric cancer), lower GI disease (diverticulosis, colonic polyps, colon carcinoma, inflammatory bowel disease, vascular ectasias, hemorrhoids).	Although fecal occult blood testing is an accepted screening test for colon carcinoma, the sensitivity and specificity of the test are low, and screening has not yet been shown to reduce mortality. An asymptomatic patient > 45 years old with a positive Hemoccult II test has about a 10% chance of having colo-rectal cancer, and a high percentage of existing lesions (50–60%) will not be detected. Hemoquant is a quantitative test for fecal occult blood that is specific for heme and measures both intact and metabolized hemoglobin. It is not used routinely. Ref: Ann Intern Med 1990;112:328. Ref: JAMA 1989;261:586.
Ferritin, serum Males 16–300 Females 4–161 ng/mL [μg/L] Marbled $$	Ferritin is the body's major iron storage protein. The serum ferritin level correlates with total body iron stores. The test is used to detect iron deficiency, to monitor response to iron therapy, and, in iron overload states, to monitor iron removal therapy. It is also used to predict homozygosity for hemochromatosis in relatives of affected patients. In the absence of liver disease, it is a more sensitive test for iron deficiency than serum iron and iron-binding capacity (transferrin saturation).	**Increased in:** Iron overload (hemochromatosis, hemosiderosis), acute or chronic liver disease, alcoholism, various malignancies (eg, leukemia, Hodgkin's disease), chronic inflammatory disorders (eg, rheumatoid arthritis), transfusion, thalassemia minor. **Decreased in:** Iron deficiency.	Serum ferritin is clinically useful in distinguishing between iron deficiency anemia (serum ferritin levels diminished) and anemia of chronic disease (levels usually normal or elevated). Serum ferritin is also a good test for separating iron deficiency (low values) from thalassemia minor (normal or high values). Liver disease will increase serum ferritin levels and mask the diagnosis of iron deficiency. Ref: N Engl J Med 1974;290:1213.

	α-Fetoprotein	Fibrin D-dimers
α-Fetoprotein, serum (AFP) 0–15 ng/mL [μg/L] Marbled $$ Avoid hemolysis.	α-Fetoprotein is a glycoprotein produced both early in fetal life and by some tumors.	**Increased in:** Hepatocellular carcinoma (72%), massive hepatic necrosis (74%), viral hepatitis (34%), chronic active hepatitis (29%), cirrhosis (11%), regional enteritis (5%), benign gynecologic diseases (22%), testicular carcinoma (embryonal (70%), teratocarcinoma (64%), teratoma (37%), ovarian carcinoma (57%), endometrial cancer (50%), cervical cancer (53%), pancreatic cancer (23%), gastric cancer (18%), colon cancer (5%). **Negative in:** Seminoma.	The test is not sensitive or specific enough to be used as a general screening test. However, screening may be justified in very high risk populations for hepatocellular cancer. In hepatocellular cancer or germ cell tumors associated with elevated AFP, the test may be helpful in detecting recurrence after therapy. AFP is also used to screen pregnant women at 15–20 weeks gestation for possible fetal neural tube defects. AFP levels in maternal serum or amniotic fluid is compared with levels expected at a given gestational age. Ref: Mayo Clin Proc 1982;57:129. Ref: Lancet 1977;1:1323. Ref: N Engl J Med 1987;317:342.
Fibrin D-dimers, plasma Negative Blue $$	Plasmin acts on fibrin to form various fibrin degradation products. A monoclonal antibody is used to quantitate the D-dimer fragments.	**Increased in:** Disseminated intravascular coagulation (DIC), other thrombotic disorders, pulmonary embolism, venous or arterial thrombosis.	Fibrin D-dimer assay has replaced the Fibrin(ogen) Split Products test as a screen for DIC, because the D-dimer assay can distinguish fibrin degradation products (in DIC) from fibrinogen degradation products (in primary fibrinogenolysis). Since the presence of fibrin D-dimer is not specific for DIC, the definitive diagnosis of DIC must depend on other tests, including the platelet count and serum fibrinogen level. Ref: Am J Clin Pathol 1986;85:360.

Test/Range/Collection	Physiologic Basis	Interpretation (sensitivity)	Comments
Fibrinogen (functional), plasma 175–433 mg/dL [1.75–4.3 g/L] *Panic:* < 75 mg/dL Blue $	Fibrinogen is synthesized in the liver and has a half-life of about 4 days. Thrombin cleaves fibrinogen to form insoluble fibrin monomers, which polymerize to form a clot.	**Increased in:** Inflammatory states (acute phase reactant), oral contraceptives, pregnancy. **Decreased in:** Decreased hepatic synthesis, increased consumption (disseminated intravascular coagulation [DIC]).	Hypofibrinogenemia is an important diagnostic laboratory feature of DIC. Ref: Blood 1982;60:284.
Fluorescent treponemal antibody-absorbed (FTA-ABS), serum Nonreactive Marbled $$	Detects specific antibodies against *Treponema pallidum.* Patient's serum is first diluted with nonpathogenic treponemal antigens (to bind nonspecific antibodies). The absorbed serum is placed on a slide that contains fixed *T pallidum.* Fluorescein-labeled antihuman gamma globulin is then added to bind to and visualize (under a fluorescence microscope) the patient's antibody on treponemes.	**Reactive in:** Syphilis: primary (95%), secondary (100%), late latent (100%); also rarely positive in collagen-vascular diseases in the presence of antinuclear antibody.	Used to confirm a reactive nontreponemal screening serologic test for syphilis such as RPR or VDRL (see p 121 and p 138, respectively). Once positive, the FTA-ABS may remain positive for life. However, a recent study found that at 36 months after treatment, 24% of patients had nonreactive FTA-ABS tests. In a study of HIV-infected men with a prior history of syphilis, 38% of patients with AIDS or ARC had loss of reactivity to treponemal tests, compared with 7% of HIV-seropositive asymptomatic men and 0% of HIV-seronegative men. Ref: Ann Intern Med 1991;114:1005. Ref: J Infect Dis 1990;162:862. Ref: Ann Intern Med 1986;104:368.

	Folic acid	Follicle-stimulating hormone
	Red cell folate level correlates better than serum folate level with tissue folate deficiency. A low red cell folate level may indicate either folate or B$_{12}$ deficiency. A therapeutic trial of folate (and not red cell or serum folate testing) is indicated when the clinical and dietary history is strongly suggestive of folate deficiency and the peripheral smear shows hypersegmented polymorphonuclear leukocytes. However, the possibility of vitamin B$_{12}$ deficiency must always be considered in the setting of megaloblastic anemia, since folate therapy will treat the hematologic, but not the neurologic, sequelae of vitamin B$_{12}$ deficiency. Ref: Blood 1983;61:624.	Test indicated in the workup of amenorrhea in women (see Amenorrhea algorithm, p 251), delayed puberty, impotence, and infertility in men. Ref: Br Med J 1987;294:815.
	Decreased in: Tissue folate deficiency (from dietary folate deficiency), B$_{12}$ deficiency (50–60%, since cellular uptake of folate depends on B$_{12}$).	**Increased in:** Primary (ovarian) gonadal failure, ovarian or testicular agenesis, castration, postmenopause, Klinefelter's syndrome, drugs. **Decreased in:** Hypothalamic disorders, pituitary disorders, pregnancy, anorexia nervosa. Drugs: corticosteroids, oral contraceptives.
	Folate is a vitamin necessary for methyl group transfer in thymidine formation, and hence DNA synthesis. Deficiency can result in megaloblastic anemia.	FSH is stimulated by the hypothalamic hormone GnRH and is then secreted from the anterior pituitary in a pulsatile fashion. Levels rise during the preovulatory phase of the menstrual cycle and then decline.
Folic acid (RBC), whole blood 165–760 ng/mL [370–1720 nmol/L] Lavender $$$		**Follicle-stimulating hormone**, serum (FSH) Female: 2–15 Peak production: 20–50 Male: 1–10 mIU/mL [IU/L] (laboratory-specific) Marbled $$

Test/Range/Collection	Physiologic Basis	Interpretation (sensitivity)	Comments
Free erythrocyte protoporphyrin, whole blood (FEP) < 35 µg/dL (method-dependent) Lavender $$$	Protoporphyrin is produced in the next to last step of heme synthesis. In the last step, iron is incorporated into protoporphyrin to produce heme. Enzyme deficiencies, lack of iron, or presence of interfering substances (lead) can disrupt this process and cause elevated FEP.	**Increased in:** Decreased iron incorporation into heme (iron deficiency, infection, and lead poisoning), erythropoietic protoporphyria.	FEP can be used to screen for lead poisoning in children provided that iron deficiency has been ruled out. Test does not discriminate between uroporphyrin, coproporphyrin, and protoporphyrin, but protoporphyrin is the predominant porphyrin measured. Ref: Clin Pediatrics 1991;30:74.
Gamma-glutamyl transpeptidase, serum (GGT) 9–85 U/L [0.15–1.42 µkat/L] (laboratory-specific) Marbled $	GGT is an enzyme present in liver, kidney, and pancreas. It transfers C-terminal glutamic acid from a peptide to other peptides of L-amino acids. It is induced by alcohol intake and is an extremely sensitive indicator of liver disease, particularly alcoholic liver disease.	**Increased in:** Liver disease: acute viral or toxic hepatitis, chronic or subacute hepatitis, alcoholic hepatitis, cirrhosis, biliary tract obstruction (intrahepatic or extrahepatic), primary or metastatic liver neoplasm, mononucleosis. Drugs (by enzyme induction): phenytoin, barbiturates, alcohol.	GGT is useful in follow-up of alcoholics undergoing treatment since the test is sensitive to modest alcohol intake. Test is positive in 90% of patients with liver disease. GGT is used to confirm hepatic origin of elevated serum alkaline phosphatase. Ref: Dig Dis Sci 1988;33:1601.

	Gastrin	Glucose
Gastrin, serum < 300 pg/mL [ng/L] Marbled $$ Overnight fasting required.	Gastrin is secreted from G cells in the stomach antrum and stimulates acid secretion from the gastric parietal cells. Values fluctuate throughout the day but are lowest in the early morning.	**Increased in:** Gastrinoma (Zollinger-Ellison syndrome) (93%), antral G cell hyperplasia, hypochlorhydria, achlorhydria, chronic atrophic gastritis, pernicious anemia. Drugs: antacids, cimetidine, and other H_2 blockers. **Decreased in:** Antrectomy with vagotomy.	Gastrin is the first-line test for determining whether a patient with active ulcer disease has a gastrinoma. Gastric analysis is not indicated. Before interpreting an elevated level, be sure that the patient is not taking antacids or H_2 blockers. Ref: Mayo Clin Proc 1982;57:211. Ref: Ann Intern Med 1983;98:59.
Glucose, serum 60–115 mg/dL [3.3–6.3 mmol/L] **Panic:** < 40 or > 500 mg/dL Marbled $ Overnight fasting usually required.	Normally, the glucose concentration in extracellular fluid is closely regulated so that a source of energy is readily available to tissues and so that no glucose is excreted in the urine.	**Increased in:** Diabetes mellitus, Cushing's syndrome (10–15%), chronic pancreatitis (30%) Drugs: corticosteroids, phenytoin, estrogen, thiazides. **Decreased in:** Pancreatic islet B cell disease with increased insulin, insulinoma, adrenocortical insufficiency, hypopituitarism, diffuse liver disease, malignancy (adrenocortical, stomach, fibrosarcoma), infant of a diabetic mother, enzyme deficiency diseases (eg, galactosemia). Drugs: insulin, ethanol, propranolol; sulfonylureas, tolbutamide, and other oral hypoglycemic agents.	Diagnosis of diabetes mellitus requires a fasting plasma glucose of > 140 mg/dL on more than one occasion. Hypoglycemia is defined as a glucose of < 50 mg/dL in men and < 40 mg/dL in women. Ref: Mayo Clin Proc 1985;60:844. Ref: N Engl J Med 1976;294:766.

	Glucose tolerance test		
Test/Range/Collection	**Physiologic Basis**	**Interpretation (sensitivity)**	**Comments**
Glucose tolerance test, serum Fasting: < 115 1-hour: < 200 2-hour: < 140 mg/dL [Fasting: < 6.4 1-hour: < 11.0 2-hour: < 7.7 mmol/L] Marbled $$ Subjects should receive a 150–200 g/day carbohydrate diet for at least 3 days prior to test. A 75 g glucose dose is dissolved in 300 mL of water for adults (1.75 g/kg for children) and given after an overnight fast. Serial determinations of plasma or serum venous blood glucoses are obtained at baseline, at 1 hour, and at 2 hours.	The test determines the ability of a patient to respond appropriately to a glucose load.	**Increased glucose rise (decreased glucose tolerance) in:** Diabetes mellitus, impaired glucose tolerance, gestational diabetes, severe liver disease, hyperthyroidism, stress (infection), increased absorption of glucose from GI tract (hyperthyroidism, gastrectomy, gastroenterostomy, vagotomy, excess glucose intake), Cushing's syndrome, pheochromocytoma. Drugs: diuretics, oral contraceptives, glucocorticoids, nicotinic acid, phenytoin. **Decreased glucose rise (flat glucose curve) in:** Intestinal disease (celiac sprue, Whipple's disease), adrenal insufficiency (Addison's disease), hypopituitarism), pancreatic islet cell tumors, or hyperplasia.	Test is not generally required for diagnosis of diabetes mellitus; diagnosis is made by finding fasting plasma glucose levels of > 140 mg/dL on more than one occasion. In screening for gestational diabetes, the glucose tolerance test is performed between 24 and 28 weeks of gestation. After a 50 g oral glucose load, a 2-hour postprandial blood glucose is measured as a screen. If the result is > 140 mg/dL, then the full test with 100 g glucose load is done using the following reference ranges: Fasting: < 105 1-hour: < 190 2-hour: < 165 3-hour: < 145 mg/dL Ref: Annu Rev Med 1983;34:295.

	G6PD screen	Glutamine
Glucose-6-phosphate dehydrogenase screen, whole blood (G6PD) 4–8 U/g Hb [0.07–0.14 µkat/L] Green or blue $$	G6PD is an enzyme in the hexose monophosphate shunt that is essential in generating reduced glutathione and NADPH, which protect hemoglobin from oxidative denaturation. Numerous G6PD isoenzymes have been identified. Most African-Americans have G6PD-A(+) isoenzyme. 10–15% have G6PD-A(–), which has only 15% of normal enzyme activity. It is transmitted in an X-linked recessive manner. Some Mediterranean people have the B– variant that has extremely low enzyme activity (1% of normal).	**Increased in:** Young erythrocytes (reticulocytosis). **Decreased in:** G6PD deficiency.	In deficient patients, hemolytic anemia can be triggered by oxidant agents: antimalarial drugs (eg, chloroquine), nalidixic acid, nitrofurantoin, phenacetin, vitamin C, and some sulfonamides. Any African-American about to be given an oxidant drug should be screened for G6PD deficiency. (Also screen people from certain Mediterranean areas: Sardinia, Greece, Italy, etc.) Hemolytic episodes can also occur in deficient patients who eat fava beans, in patients with diabetic acidosis, and in infections. G6PD deficiency may be the cause of hemolytic disease of newborns in Asians and Mediterraneans. Ref: Ann Intern Med 1985;103:245. Ref: Br J Haematol 1979;43:465.
Glutamine, CSF 6–15 mg/dL *Panic:* > 40 mg/dL $$$ Collect CSF in a plastic tube.	Glutamine is synthesized in the brain from ammonia and glutamic acid. Elevated CSF glutamine levels are associated with hepatic encephalopathy.	**Increased in:** Hepatic encephalopathy.	Test is not indicated if albumin, alanine aminotransferase (ALT), bilirubin, and alkaline phosphatase are normal or if there is no clinical evidence of liver disease. Hepatic encephalopathy is essentially ruled out if the CSF glutamine is normal. Ref: Arch Intern Med 1971;127:1033. Ref: Science 1974;183:81.

Test/Range/Collection	Physiologic Basis	Interpretation (sensitivity)	Comments
Glycated (Glycosylated) hemoglobin, serum (HbA$_{1c}$) 3.9–6.9% (method-dependent) Lavender $$	During the life span of each red blood cell, glucose combines with hemoglobin to produce a stable glycated hemoglobin. The level of glycated hemoglobin is related to the mean plasma glucose level during the prior 1–3 months. It is used to monitor long-term control of blood glucose level.	**Increased in:** Diabetes mellitus, splenectomy. Falsely high results can occur depending on the method used and may be due to presence of hemoglobin F or uremia. **Decreased in:** Any condition that shortens red cell life span (hemolytic anemias, congenital spherocytosis, sickle cell disease, hemoglobinopathies).	Test is not indicated for diagnosis of diabetes mellitus. There are 3 glycated A hemoglobins, HbA$_{1a}$, HbA$_{1b}$ and HbA$_{1c}$. Some assays quantitate HbA$_{1c}$; some quantitate total HbA$_1$; and some quantitate all glycated hemoglobins, not just A. Reference ranges and spurious results (including variability based on storage, temperature, and pH conditions) are method-specific. Ref: J Clin Chem Clin Biochem 1988; 26:809. Ref: Ann Intern Med 1984;101:710. Ref: N Engl J Med 1984;310:341.
Growth hormone, serum (GH) 0–5 ng/mL [μg/L] Marbled $$$	Growth hormone is a single-chain polypeptide of 191 amino acids that induces the generation of somatomedins, which directly stimulate collagen and protein synthesis. GH levels are subject to wide fluctuations during the day.	**Increased in:** Acromegaly (80% have GH levels > 10 ng/mL), Laron dwarfism (defective GH receptor), starvation. Drugs: dopamine, levodopa. **Decreased in:** Pituitary dwarfism, hypopituitarism.	Nonsuppressibility of GH levels to < 2 ng/mL after 100 g oral glucose and elevation of somatomedin C levels are the 2 most sensitive tests for acromegaly. Random determinations of GH are rarely useful in the diagnosis of acromegaly. For the diagnosis of hypopituitarism or growth hormone deficiency in children, an insulin hypoglycemia test has been used. Failure to increase GH levels to > 5 ng/mL after insulin (0.1 U/kg) is consistent with GH deficiency. Ref: N Engl J Med 1991;324:826. Ref: Hosp Pract 1978;13(Aug):57.

	Haptoglobin	Hematocrit	Hemoglobin A$_2$
	Low haptoglobin is considered an indicator of hemolysis, but it is of uncertain clinical predictive value because of the greater prevalence of other conditions associated with low levels and because of occasional normal individuals who have very low levels. It thus has low specificity. High-normal levels probably rule out significant intravascular hemolysis. Ref: JAMA 1980;243:1909.	Conversion from hemoglobin (Hb) to hematocrit is roughly Hb × 3 = Hct. Hematocrit reported by clinical laboratories is not a spun hematocrit. The spun hematocrit may be spuriously high if the centrifuge is not calibrated, if the specimen is not spun to constant volume, or if there is "trapped plasma." Ref: JAMA 1988;259:2433.	Test is useful in the diagnosis of β-thalassemia minor (in absence of iron deficiency, which decreases HbA$_2$ and can mask the diagnosis). Ref: Blood 1988;72:1107.
	Increased in: Acute and chronic infection (acute phase reactant), malignancy, biliary obstruction, ulcerative colitis, myocardial infarction, and diabetes mellitus. **Decreased in:** Newborns and children, posttransfusion intravascular hemolysis, autoimmune hemolytic anemia, liver disease (10%). May be decreased following uneventful transfusion (10%) for unknown reasons.	**Increased in:** Hemoconcentration (as in dehydration, burns, vomiting), polycythemia, extreme physical exercise. **Decreased in:** *Macrocytic anemia* (liver disease, hypothyroidism, vitamin B$_{12}$ deficiency, folate deficiency), *normocytic anemia* (early iron deficiency, anemia of chronic disease, hemolytic anemia, acute hemorrhage) and *microcytic anemia* (iron deficiency, thalassemia).	**Increased in:** β-Thalassemia major (HbA$_2$ levels 4–10% of total Hb), β-thalassemia minor (HbA$_2$ levels 4–8% of total Hb). **Decreased in:** Untreated iron deficiency, hemoglobin H disease.
	Haptoglobin is a glycoprotein synthesized in the liver that binds free hemoglobin.	The hematocrit represents the percentage of whole blood volume composed of erythrocytes. Laboratory instruments calculate the Hct from the erythrocyte count (RBC) and the mean corpuscular volume (MCV) by the formula: Hct = RBC × MCV.	HbA$_2$ is a minor component of normal adult hemoglobin (< 3.5% of total Hb).
	Haptoglobin, serum 46–316 mg/dL [0.5–3.2 g/L] Marbled $$	**Hematocrit,** whole blood (Hct) Male: 39–49% Female: 35–45% (age-dependent) Lavender $	**Hemoglobin A$_2$,** whole blood (HbA$_2$) 1.5–3.5% of total hemoglobin (Hb) Lavender $$

Test/Range/Collection	Physiologic Basis	Interpretation (sensitivity)	Comments
Hemoglobin electrophoresis, whole blood HbA: > 95 HbA$_2$: 1.5–3.5% Lavender, blue, or green $$	Hemoglobin electrophoresis is used as a screening test. It is used to detect and differentiate hemoglobin variants. Separation of hemoglobins by electrophoresis is based on different rates of migration of charged hemoglobin molecules in an electric field.	↑**HbS:** HbA > HbS = Sickle cell trait (HbAS) or sickle α-thalassemia; HbS and F, no HbA = Sickle cell anemia (HbSS) or sickle β-thalassemia; HbS > HbA and F: Sickle β⁺-thalassemia. ↑**HbC:** HbA > HbC = HbC trait (HbAC); HbC and F, no HbA = HbC disease; HbC > HbA = HbC β⁺-thalassemia. ↑**HbH:** HbH disease. ↑**HbA$_2$, F:** See HbA$_2$, above, and HbF, below.	Evaluation of a suspected hemoglobinopathy should include electrophoresis of a hemolysate to detect an abnormal hemoglobin and quantitation of hemoglobin A$_2$ and F. Ref: Semin Perinatol 1990;14:483.
Hemoglobin, fetal, whole blood (HbF) Adult: < 2% (varies with age) Lavender, blue, or green $$	Fetal hemoglobin constitutes about 75% of total hemoglobin at birth and declines to 50% at 6 weeks, 5% at 6 months, and < 1.5% by 1 year. During the first year, adult hemoglobin (HbA) becomes the predominant hemoglobin.	**Increased in:** Hereditary disorders: eg, β-thalassemia major (60–100% of total Hb is HbF), β-thalassemia minor (2–5% HbF), sickle cell anemia (1–3% HbF), hereditary persistence of fetal hemoglobin (10–40% HbF). Acquired disorders (< 10% HbF): aplastic anemia, megaloblastic anemia, leukemia. **Decreased in:** Hemolytic anemia of the newborn.	Semiquantitative acid elution test provides an estimate of fetal hemoglobin only and varies widely between laboratories. Useful in distinguishing hereditary persistence of fetal hemoglobin (all RBCs show an increase in fetal hemoglobin) from β-thalassemia minor (only a portion of RBCs are affected). Enzyme-linked antiglobulin test is used to detect fetal red cells in the Rh(−) maternal circulation in suspected cases of Rh sensitization and to determine the amount of RhoGAM to administer (1 vial/15 mL fetal RBC). Ref: J Clin Pathol 1972;25:738.

	Hemoglobin	Hemosiderin
Hemoglobin, total, whole blood (Hb) Male: 13.6–17.5 Female: 12.0–15.5 g/dL (age-dependent) [Male: 136–175 Female: 120–155 g/L] ***Panic:*** ≤ 7 g/dL Lavender $	Hemoglobin is the major protein of erythrocytes and transports oxygen from the lungs to peripheral tissues. It is measured by spectrophotometry on automated instruments after hemolysis of red cells and conversion of all hemoglobin to cyanmethemoglobin.	**Increased in:** Hemoconcentration (as in dehydration, burns, vomiting), polycythemia, extreme physical exercise, heavy smoking (due to presence of nonfunctional carboxyhemoglobin). **Decreased in:** *Macrocytic anemia* (liver disease, hypothyroidism, vitamin B_{12} deficiency, folate deficiency), *normocytic anemia* (early iron deficiency, anemia of chronic disease, hemolytic anemia, acute hemorrhage) and *microcytic anemia* (iron deficiency, thalassemia). Hypertriglyceridemia and very high white blood cell counts can cause false elevations of Hb. Ref: JAMA 1988;259:2433.
Hemosiderin, urine Negative Urine container $$ Fresh, random sample.	Hemosiderin is a protein produced by the digestion of hemoglobin. Its presence in the urine indicates acute or chronic release of free hemoglobin into the circulation with accompanying depletion of the scavenging proteins, hemopexin and haptoglobin. Presence of hemosiderin usually indicates intravascular hemolysis or recent transfusion.	**Increased in:** Intravascular hemolysis: hemolytic transfusion reactions, paroxysmal nocturnal hemoglobinuria, microangiopathic hemolytic anemia, mechanical destruction of erythrocytes (heart valve hemolysis), sickle cell anemia, thalassemia major, oxidant drugs with G6PD deficiency (eg, dapsone). Hemochromatosis. Ref: J Lab Clin Med 1951;38:3.

Test/Range/Collection	Physiologic Basis	Interpretation (sensitivity)	Comments
Hepatitis A antibody, serum (Anti-HAV) Negative Marbled $$	Hepatitis A is caused by a nonenveloped 27 nm RNA virus of the enterovirus/picornavirus group and is usually acquired by the fecal-oral route. IgM antibody is detectable within a week after symptoms develop and persists for 6 months. IgG develops later than IgM and persists for years (see Figure 9–4, p 264, for time course of serologic changes).	**Positive in:** Acute hepatitis A (IgM), convalescence from hepatitis A (IgG).	The most commonly used test for hepatitis A antibody is an immunoassay that detects total IgG and IgM antibodies. This test can be used to establish immune status. Specific IgM testing is necessary to diagnose acute hepatitis A. IgG antibody positivity is found in 40–50% of adult population in USA and Europe (higher rates in developing nations). Ref: Mayo Clin Proc 1979;54:721.
Hepatitis B surface antigen, serum (HBsAg) Negative Marbled $$	In hepatitis B virus infection, surface antigen is detectable 2–5 weeks before onset of symptoms, rises in titer, and peaks at about the time of onset of clinical illness. Generally it persists for 1–5 months, declining in titer and disappearing with resolution of clinical symptoms (see Figure 9–5, p 265, for time course of serologic changes.).	**Increased in:** Acute hepatitis B, chronic hepatitis B (persistence of HBsAg for > 6 months, positive HBcAb [total]). HBsAg-positive carriers. May be undetectable in acute hepatitis B infection. If clinical suspicion is high, HBcAb (IgM) test is then indicated.	First-line test for the diagnosis of acute or chronic hepatitis B. If positive, no other test is needed. HBeAg is a marker of extensive viral replication found only in HBsAg-positive sera. Persistently HBeAg-positive patients are more infectious than HBeAg-negative patients and more likely to develop chronic liver disease. Ref: Annu Rev Med 1981;32:1.
Hepatitis B surface antibody, serum (HBsAb, anti-HBs) Negative Marbled $$	Test detects antibodies to hepatitis B virus (HBV) which are thought to confer immunity to hepatitis B. Since several subtypes of hepatitis B exist, there is a possibility of subsequent infection with a second subtype.	**Increased in:** Hepatitis B immunity due to HBV infection or hepatitis B vaccination. **Absent in:** Hepatitis B carrier state, nonexposure.	Test indicates immune status. It is not useful for the evaluation of acute or chronic hepatitis. (See Figure 9–5, p 265, for time course of serologic changes.) Ref: Ann Intern Med 1985;103:201. Ref: Dig Dis Sci 1986;31:620.

Test / Cost	Physiologic Basis	Interpretation	Comments
Hepatitis B core antibody, total, serum (HBcAb, anti-HBc) Negative Marbled $$	HBcAb (IgG and IgM) will be positive (as IgM) about 2 months after exposure to hepatitis B. Its persistent positivity may reflect chronic hepatitis (IgM) or recovery (IgG). (See Figure 9–5, p 265, for time course of serologic changes.)	**Positive in:** Hepatitis B (acute and chronic), hepatitis B carriers (high levels), prior hepatitis B (immune levels) when IgG present in low titer with or without HBsAb. **Negative:** After hepatitis B vaccination.	**Hepatitis B core antibody** HBcAb (total) is useful in evaluation of acute or chronic hepatitis only if HBsAg is negative. An HBcAb (IgM) test is then indicated only if the HBcAb (total) is positive. HBcAb (IgM) may be the only serologic indication of acute HBV infection. Ref: Dig Dis Sci 1985;30:1022. Ref: Mayo Clin Proc 1988;63:201.
Hepatitis C antibody, serum (HCAb) Negative Marbled $$	Detects antibody to hepatitis C virus, a recently discovered major cause of non-A, non-B hepatitis. Current screening test (ELISA immunoassay) uses C100 antigen to detect antibody. This antibody is not protective.	**Increased in:** Acute hepatitis C (only 20–50%; seroconversion may take 6 months or more), posttransfusion chronic non-A, non-B hepatitis (70–90%), sporadic chronic non-A, non-B hepatitis (30–80%), blood donors (0.5–1%), non-blood-donating general public (2–3%), hemophiliacs (75%), intravenous drug abusers (40–80%), hemodialysis patients (1–30%), male homosexuals (4%).	**Hepatitis C antibody** Sensitivity of current assays is 86%, specificity 99.5%. Hepatitis C remains a clinical diagnosis of exclusion. Seropositivity for hepatitis C documents previous exposure, not necessarily acute infection. Seronegativity in acute hepatitis does not exclude the diagnosis of hepatitis C. Ref: N Engl J Med 1989;321:1538.

Test/Range/Collection	Physiologic Basis	Interpretation (sensitivity)	Comments
Hepatitis D antibody, serum (Anti-HDV) Negative Marbled $$	This antibody is a marker for acute or persisting infection with the delta agent, a defective RNA virus that can only infect HBsAg-positive patients. Hepatitis B virus (HBV) plus hepatitis D virus (HDV) infection may be more severe than HBV infection alone. Antibody to HDV ordinarily persists for about 6 months following acute infection. Further persistence indicates carrier status.	**Increased in:** Hepatitis D.	Test only indicated in HBsAg-positive patients. Chronic HDV hepatitis occurs in 80–90% of HBsAg carriers who are superinfected with delta, but less than 5% of those who are coinfected with both viruses simultaneously. Ref: Ann Intern Med 1989;110:779. Ref: Hepatology 1985;5:188.
Heterophile agglutination, serum (Monospot) Negative Marbled $	Infectious mononucleosis is an acute saliva-transmitted infectious disease due to the Epstein-Barr virus (EBV). Heterophile antibodies (IgM) appear in 60% of mononucleosis patients within 1–2 weeks and in 80–90% within the first month. Titers are substantially diminished by 3 months after primary infection and are not detectable by 6 months.	**Positive in:** Infectious mononucleosis (90–95%).	If heterophile is negative in the setting of hematologic and clinical evidence of illness, a repeat test in 1–2 weeks may be positive. EBV serology (anti-VCA and anti-EBNA) may also be indicated, especially in children and teenage patients who may have negative heterophile tests (see EBV antibodies, p 74). Ref: Hum Pathol 1974;5:551.

	Histoplasma precipitins	*Histoplasma*, CF
Histoplasma capsulatum precipitins, serum Negative Marbled $$	This test screens for presence of *Histoplasma* antibody by detecting precipitin "H" and "M" bands. Positive H band indicates active infection, M band indicates acute or chronic infection or prior skin testing. Presence of both suggests active histoplasmosis.	**Positive in:** Previous chronic or acute *Histoplasma* infection, recent histoplasmin skin testing. Cross-reactions at low levels in patients with blastomycosis and coccidioidomycosis.	Test is useful as an adjunct to complement fixation test (see below) in diagnosis of systemic histoplasmosis. Ref: Rose NR et al (editors): *Manual of Clinical Laboratory Immunology.* American Society for Microbiology, 1986.
Histoplasma capsulatum complement fixation (CF) antibody, serum < 1:4 titer Marbled $$ Submit paired sera, one collected within 1 week of illness and another 2–3 weeks later. Avoid hemolysis.	Quantitates level of *Histoplasma* antibody. Antibodies in primary pulmonary infections are generally found within 4 weeks after exposure and frequently are present at the time symptoms appear.	**Increased in:** Previous, chronic, or acute *Histoplasma* infection (75–80%), recent histoplasmin skin testing (20%), other fungal disease, leishmaniasis. Cross-reactions in patients with blastomycosis and coccidioidomycosis.	Elevated CF titers are suggestive of infection. Titers of > 1:32 or rising titers are usually indicative of active infection. Histoplasmin skin test is not recommended for diagnosis since it interferes with subsequent serologic tests. Ref: Rose NR et al (editors): *Manual of Clinical Laboratory Immunology.* American Society for Microbiology, 1986.

Test/Range/Collection	Physiologic Basis	Interpretation (sensitivity)	Comments
		HIV Antibody	**HLA typing**
HIV Antibody, serum Negative Marbled $$	This test detects antibody against the human immunodeficiency virus-1 (HIV-1), the etiologic agent of AIDS. HIV antibody test is considered positive only when a repeatedly reactive enzyme immunoassay (EIA) is confirmed by a Western blot analysis or immunofluorescent antibody test (IFA).	**Positive in:** HIV infection: EIA sensitivity > 99% after first 2–4 months of infection, specificity 99%. When combined with confirmatory test, specificity is 99.995%.	A positive p24 antigen test in an HIV antibody-negative individual must be confirmed by a viral neutralization assay. While Western blot test is currently the most sensitive and specific assay for HIV serodiagnosis, it is highly dependent on the proficiency of the laboratory performing the test and on the standardization of the procedure. Ref: JAMA 1991;266:2861. Ref: Arch Pathol Lab Med 1989;113:975. Ref: Ann Intern Med 1987;106:671.
HLA typing, serum and blood (HLA) Marbled (2 mL) and Yellow (40 mL) $$$$ Specimens must be < 24 hours old. Refrigerate serum, but not yellow tubes.	The human leukocyte antigen (HLA) system consists of 4 closely linked loci (HLA-A, -B, -C, and -DR) located on the short arm of chromosome 6. In HLA typing, peripheral blood lymphocytes are used to test the compatibility of antigens in donor and recipient cells.	**Useful in:** Evaluation of transplant candidates and potential donors to determine compatibility; paternity and forensic testing.	While diseases associated with particular HLA antigens have been identified, HLA typing for the diagnosis of these diseases is not generally indicated. Ref: Cell 1984;36:1.

	HLA-B27 typing	5-HIAA	IgG index
HLA-B27 typing, whole blood Negative Yellow $$$ Specimens must be < 24 hours old.	The HLA-B27 allele is found in approximately 8% of the US white population. It occurs less frequently in the African-American population.	There is an increased incidence of spondyloarthritis among patients who are HLA-B27-positive. HLA-B27 is present in 88% of patients with ankylosing spondylitis. It is also associated with the development of Reiter's syndrome (80%) following infection with *Shigella* or *Salmonella*.	The best diagnostic test for ankylosing spondylitis is a lumbar spine film and not HLA-B27 typing. HLA-B27 testing is not usually clinically indicated. Ref: Ann Intern Med 1980;92:208.
5-Hydroxy-indoleacetic acid, urine (5-HIAA) 2–8 mg/24 h [10–40 µmol/d] Urine bottle containing hydrochloric acid $$	Serotonin (5-hydroxytryptamine) is a neurotransmitter that is metabolized by monoamine oxidase (MAO) to 5-HIAA and then excreted into the urine. Serotonin is secreted by most carcinoid tumors, which arise from neuroendocrine cells in locations derived from the embryonic gut.	**Increased in:** Metastatic carcinoid tumor (foregut, midgut, and bronchial). Nontropical sprue (slight increase). Diet of bananas, walnuts, avocado, eggplant, pineapple, plums. Drugs: reserpine. **Negative in:** Rectal carcinoids (usually), renal insufficiency. Drugs: MAO inhibitors, phenothiazines.	Since most carcinoid tumors drain into the portal vein and serotonin is rapidly cleared by the liver, the carcinoid syndrome (flushing, bronchial constriction, diarrhea, hypotension, and cardiac valvular lesions) is a late manifestation of carcinoid tumors, appearing only after hepatic metastasis has occurred. Ref: N Engl J Med 1986;315:702.
IgG index, serum and CSF 0.29–0.59 ratio Marbled and glass/plastic tube for CSF $$$ Collect serum and CSF simultaneously.	This test compares CSF IgG and albumin levels to serum levels. An increased ratio allegedly reflects synthesis of IgG within the central nervous system. IgG index = $$\dfrac{CSF\ IgG\,/\,CSF\ albumin}{serum\ IgG\,/\,serum\ albumin}$$	**Increased in:** Multiple sclerosis (80–90%), neurosyphilis, subacute sclerosing panencephalitis, other inflammatory and infectious diseases.	Test is reasonably sensitive but not specific for multiple sclerosis. (Compare with Oligoclonal bands, p 109.) Ref: Mayo Clin Proc 1989;64:577. Ref: Ann Neurol 1980;8:426.

Test/Range/Collection	Physiologic Basis	Interpretation (sensitivity)	Comments
	Immunoelectrophoresis		**Immunoglobulins**
Immunoelectrophoresis (IEP), serum Negative Marbled $$$	Immunoelectrophoresis is used to identify specific immunoglobulin (Ig) classes. Serum is separated electrophoretically and reacted with antisera of known specificity. Newer technique (immunofixation) is available.	**Positive in:** Presence of identifiable monoclonal paraprotein. The most common form of myeloma is the IgG type.	Test is indicated to identify an Ig spike seen on serum protein electrophoresis, to differentiate a polyclonal from a monoclonal increase, and to identify the nature of a monoclonal increase. Test is not quantitative and is not sensitive enough to use for the evaluation of immunodeficiency. Order quantitative immunoglobulins for this purpose (see below). Ref: Clin Lab Med 1986;6:403,601.
Immunoglobulins, serum (Ig) IgA: 78–367 IgG: 583–1761 IgM: 52–335 mg/dL [IgA: 0.78–3.67 IgG: 5.83–17.6 IgM: 0.52–3.35 g/L] Marbled $$$	IgG makes up about 85% of total serum immunoglobulins and predominates late in immune responses. It is the only immunoglobulin to cross the placenta. IgM antibody predominates early in immune responses. Secretory IgA plays an important role in host defense mechanisms by blocking transport of microbes across mucosal surfaces.	↑**IgG:** *Polyclonal:* Autoimmune diseases (eg, SLE, rheumatoid arthritis), sarcoidosis, chronic liver diseases, some parasitic diseases, chronic or recurrent infections. *Monoclonal:* Multiple myeloma (IgG type), lymphomas, or other malignancies. ↑**IgM:** *Polyclonal:* Isolated infections such as viral hepatitis, infectious mononucleosis, early response to bacterial or parasitic infection. *Monoclonal:* Waldenström's macroglobulinemia, lymphoma. ↑**IgA:** *Polyclonal:* Chronic liver disease, chronic infections (especially of the GI and respiratory tracts). *Monoclonal:* Multiple myeloma (IgA). ↓**IgG:** Immunosuppressive therapy, genetic (severe combined immunodeficiency, Wiskott-Aldrich syndrome, common variable immunodeficiency). ↓**IgM:** Immunosuppressive therapy. ↓**IgA:** Inherited IgA deficiency (ataxia-telangiectasia, combined immunodeficiency disorders).	Quantitative immunoglobulin levels are indicated in the evaluation of immunodeficiency or the quantitation of a paraprotein. IgG deficiency is associated with recurrent and occasionally severe pyogenic infections. The most common form of multiple myeloma is the IgG type. Ref: Science 1986;231:1241.

	Inhibitor screen	Insulin antibodies	Insulin
Test / specimen	**Inhibitor screen,** plasma Negative Blue $$ Fill tube completely.	**Insulin antibodies,** serum Negative Marbled $$$	**Insulin, immunoreactive,** serum 6–35 µU/mL [42–243 pmol/L] Marbled $$ Fasting sample required. Measure glucose concurrently.
Interpretation	**Positive in:** Presence of inhibitor (lupus anticoagulant or factor-specific antibodies). **Negative in:** Factor deficiencies.	**Increased in:** Insulin therapy, type I diabetics before treatment (secondary to autoimmune pancreatic B cell destruction).	**Increased in:** Insulin-resistant states (eg, obesity, type II diabetes mellitus, uremia, glucocorticoids, acromegaly), liver disease, surreptitious use of insulin or oral hypoglycemic agents, insulinoma (pancreatic islet cell tumor). **Decreased in:** Type I diabetes mellitus, hypopituitarism.
Comments	Test is useful for evaluating a prolonged partial thromboplastin time (PTT), prothrombin time (PT), or thrombin time. (Presence of heparin should first be excluded.) Patient's plasma is mixed with normal plasma and a PTT is performed. If the patient has a factor deficiency, the postmixing PTT will be normal. If an inhibitor is present, it will be prolonged. Lupus anticoagulant prolongs a PTT immediately. Poor sensitivity for lupus anticoagulant owing to relatively high phospholipid levels in this assay system. 1–4 hour incubation period may be needed to detect factor-specific antibodies with low in vitro affinities. Ref: Semin Thromb Hemost 1975;1:336.	Insulin antibodies develop in nearly all diabetics treated with insulin. Most antibodies are IgG and do not cause clinical problems. Occasionally, high-affinity antibodies can bind to exogenous insulin and cause insulin resistance. Insulin antibodies interfere with most assays for insulin. Insulin antibodies test is not sensitive or specific for the detection of surreptitious insulin use; use C-peptide level (see p 56). Ref: Diabetes Care 1989;12:641. Ref: Diabetic Med 1991;8:97.	Measures levels of insulin, either endogenous or exogenous. Measurement of serum insulin level has little clinical value except in the diagnosis of fasting hypoglycemia. An insulin-to-glucose ratio of > 0.3 is presumptive evidence of insulinoma. C-peptide should be used as well as serum insulin to distinguish insulinoma from surreptitious insulin use, since C-peptide will be absent with exogenous insulin use (see C-peptide, p 56). Ref: Mayo Clin Proc 1976;51:417.

Test/Range/Collection	Physiologic Basis	Interpretation (sensitivity)	Comments
			Iron	Iron-binding capacity
Iron, serum (Fe^{2+}) 50–175 µg/dL [9–31 µmol/L] Marbled $ Avoid hemolysis.	Plasma iron concentration is determined by absorption from the intestine; storage in the liver, spleen, bone marrow; rate of breakdown or loss of hemoglobin; and rate of synthesis of new hemoglobin.	**Increased in:** Hemosiderosis (eg, multiple transfusions, excess iron administration), hemolytic anemia, pernicious anemia, aplastic or hypoplastic anemia, viral hepatitis, lead poisoning, thalassemia, hemochromatosis. Drugs: estrogens, ethanol, oral contraceptives. **Decreased in:** Iron deficiency, nephrotic syndrome, chronic renal failure, many infections, active hematopoiesis, remission of pernicious anemia, hypothyroidism, malignancy (carcinoma), postoperative state, kwashiorkor, some drugs.	Test is used in evaluation of iron deficiency (see Iron-binding capacity, below and Ferritin, p 78). Ref: J Nutr 1988;118:1110. Ref: Am J Med 1964;37:62.
Iron-binding capacity, total, serum (TIBC) 250–460 µg/dL [45–82 µmol/L] Marbled $$	Iron is transported in plasma complexed to transferrin, which is synthesized in the liver. Total iron-binding capacity is calculated from transferrin levels measured immunologically. Each molecule of transferrin has two iron-binding sites, so its iron-binding capacity is 1.47 mg/g. Normally, transferrin carries an amount of iron representing about 16–60% of its capacity to bind iron (ie, % saturation of iron-binding capacity is 16–60%).	**Increased in:** Iron deficiency anemia, late pregnancy, infancy, hepatitis. Drugs: oral contraceptives. **Decreased in:** Hypoproteinemic states (eg, nephrotic syndrome, starvation, malnutrition, cancer), chronic inflammatory disorders, chronic liver disease, other chronic disease.	Increased % transferrin saturation with iron is seen in iron overload (iron poisoning, hemolytic anemia, sideroblastic anemia, thalassemia, hemochromatosis, pyridoxine deficiency, aplastic anemia). Decreased % transferrin saturation with iron is seen in iron deficiency (usually saturation < 16%). Transferrin levels can also be used to assess nutritional status. Ref: Am J Clin Pathol 1990;93:240. Ref: Am J Clin Nutr 1981;34:1600.

Test	Physiology	Interpretation	Comments
Lactate dehydrogenase, serum (LDH) 88–230 U/L [1.46–3.82 µkat/L] (laboratory-specific) Marbled $ Hemolyzed specimens are unacceptable.	LDH is an enzyme that catalyzes the interconversion of lactate and pyruvate in the presence of NAD/NADH. It is widely distributed in body cells and fluids. Because LDH is highly concentrated in red blood cells (RBCs), spuriously elevated serum levels will occur if RBCs are hemolyzed during specimen collection.	**Increased in:** Tissue necrosis, especially in acute injury of cardiac muscle, RBCs, kidney, skeletal muscle, liver, lung, or skin. Commonly elevated in various carcinomas and in *Pneumocystis carinii* pneumonia and B cell lymphoma in AIDS. Marked elevations occur in hemolytic anemias, vitamin B_{12} deficiency anemia, folate deficiency anemia, polycythemia vera, hepatitis, cirrhosis, obstructive jaundice, renal disease, musculoskeletal disease, CHF. Drugs causing hepatotoxicity or hemolysis. **Decreased in:** Drugs: clofibrate, fluoride (low dose).	LDH is elevated after myocardial infarction (for 2–7 days), in liver congestion (eg, in CHF); and in *Pneumocystis carinii* pneumonia. LDH is not a useful liver function test, and it is not specific enough for the diagnosis of hemolytic or megaloblastic anemias. Its main diagnostic use is in myocardial infarction, when the creatine kinase-MB elevation has passed (see Figure 9–6, p 266). With the availability of specific LDH$_1$ measurements, the total LDH level may no longer be useful (see LDH isoenzymes, below). Ref: Am Rev Respir Dis 1988;137:796. Ref: Clin Biochem 1990;23:375.
Lactate dehydrogenase isoenzymes, serum (LDH isoenzymes) LDH$_1$/LDH$_2$: < 0.85 Marbled $$ Hemolyzed specimens are unacceptable.	LDH consists of 5 isoenzymes separable by electrophoresis. The fraction with the greatest electrophoretic mobility is called LDH$_1$, the one with the least, LDH$_5$. LDH$_1$ is found in high concentrations in heart muscle, RBCs, and kidney cortex; isoenzyme 5, in skeletal muscle and liver.	**Increased in:** LDH$_1$/LDH$_2$ > 0.85 in myocardial infarction, hemolysis (hemolytic or megaloblastic anemia) or acute renal infarction. LDH$_5$ is increased in liver disease, congestive heart failure, skeletal muscle injury.	The only clinical indication for LDH isoenzyme measurement is to rule out myocardial infarction (flipped LDH ratio, [ie, LDH$_1$ > LDH$_2$] is usually present within 12–48 hours). Ref: Clin Chem 1980;26:1241. Ref: Ann Clin Lab Sci 1982;12:408. Ref: Hum Pathol 1984;15:706.

Test/Range/Collection	Physiologic Basis	Interpretation (sensitivity)	Comments
Lactic acid, venous blood 0.5–2.0 meq/L [mmol/L] Gray $$ Collect on ice in gray tube containing fluoride to inhibit in vitro glycolysis and lactic acid production.	Severe tissue anoxia leads to anaerobic glucose metabolism with production of lactic acid.	**Increased in:** Lactic acidosis, ethanol ingestion, sepsis, shock, liver disease, diabetic ketoacidosis, muscular exercise, hypoxia; prolonged use of a tourniquet (spurious elevation); type I glycogen storage disease, fructose 1,6-diphosphatase deficiency (rare). Drugs: phenformin, isoniazid toxicity.	Lactic acidosis should be suspected when there is a markedly increased anion gap (> 18 meq/L) in the absence of other causes (eg, renal failure, ketosis, ethanol, methanol, or salicylate). Ref: N Engl J Med 1974;291:773.
Lead, whole blood (Pb) Child: < 25 Adult: < 40 μg/dL [Child: < 1.21 Adult: < 1.93 μmol/L] Navy $$ Use trace metal-free navy blue top tube with heparin.	Lead salts are absorbed through ingestion, inhalation, or the skin. About 5–10% of ingested lead is found in blood and 95% of this is in erythrocytes. 80–90% is taken up by bone, where it is relatively inactive. Lead poisons enzymes by binding to protein disulfide groups, leading to cell death. Lead levels fluctuate. Several specimens may be needed to rule out lead poisoning.	**Increased in:** Lead poisoning, including abnormal ingestion (especially lead-containing paint, moonshine whiskey), occupational exposures (metal smelters, miners, welders, storage battery builders, ship manufacturers, auto manufacturers, printing workers, pottery workers, gasoline refinery workers), retained bullets.	Blood lead levels are useful in the diagnosis of acute lead poisoning. Subtle neurologic impairment may be detectable in children with lead levels of 15 μg/dL and in adults at 30 μg/dL; full-blown symptoms appear at > 60 μg/dL. Industrial limit: < 50 μg/dL. Ref: Medicine 1983;62:221.

Test / Specimen / Cost	Physiologic Basis	Interpretation	Comments
Lecithin/Sphingo-myelin ratio, amniotic fluid (L/S ratio) > 2.0 (method-dependent) $$$ Collect in a plastic tube.	This test is used to estimate lung maturity in fetuses at risk for hyaline membrane disease. As fetal pulmonary surfactant matures, there is a rapid rise in amniotic fluid lecithin content. To circumvent the dependency of lecithin concentrations on amniotic fluid volume and analytic recovery of lecithin, the assay examines the lecithin/sphingomyelin ratio.	**Increased in:** Contamination of amniotic fluid by blood, meconium, or vaginal secretions that contain lecithin (false-positives). **Decreased in:** Fetal lung immaturity; 40% of normal fetuses.	Test identifies fetal lung maturity effectively only 60% of the time—ie. 40% of fetuses with a L/S ratio of < 2.0 will not develop hyaline membrane disease. Precision of L/S ratio test is poor; results on a single sample may vary by ± 25%. Test is not reliable to assess fetal lung maturity in offspring of diabetic mothers. Ref: Med Decis Making 1990;10:201. Ref: Am J Clin Pathol 1983;79:52. Ref: Clin Chem 1978;24:1144.
Legionella antibody, serum < 1:32 titer Marbled $$$ Submit paired sera, one collected within 2 weeks of illness and another 2–3 weeks later.	*Legionella pneumophila* is a weakly staining gram-negative bacillus that causes Pontiac fever (acute influenza-like illness) and legionnaires' disease (a pneumonia that may progress to a severe multisystem illness). It does not grow on routine bacteriologic culture media. Antibodies are detected by indirect immunofluorescent tests to serogroup 1 of *L pneumophila*. There are at least 6 serogroups of *L pneumophila* and at least 22 species of *Legionella*.	**Increased in:** *Legionella* infection (80% of patients with pneumonia have a 4-fold rise in titer), cross-reactions with other infectious agents (*Yersinia Pestis* [plague], *Francisella tularensis* [tularemia], *Bacteroides fragilis, Mycoplasma pneumoniae,* or *Leptospira interrogans*).	A > 4-fold rise in titer to > 1:128 in specimens gathered more than 3 weeks apart indicates recent infection. A single titer of > 1:256 is considered diagnostic. About 50–60% of cases of legionellosis may have a positive direct fluorescent antibody test. Culture can have a sensitivity of 50%. All three methods may increase sensitivity to 90%. This test is species-specific. Polyvalent antiserum is needed to test for all serogroups and species. Ref: JAMA 1983;250:1981. Ref: Am Rev Respir Dis 1980;121:317.

Test/Range/Collection	Physiologic Basis	Interpretation (sensitivity)	Comments
		Leukocyte alkaline phosphatase	Leukocyte count
Leukocyte alkaline phosphatase, whole blood (LAP) 40–130 Based on 0–4+ rating of 100 PMNs Green $$ Blood smear from finger stick preferred. If collecting venous blood, make smear as soon as possible.	The test measures the amount of alkaline phosphatase in neutrophils in a semiquantitative fashion. Neutrophilic leukocytes on a peripheral blood smear are stained for alkaline phosphatase activity and then 100 are scored on a scale from 0 to 4+ on the basis of the intensity of the dye in their cytoplasm.	**Increased in:** Leukemoid reaction (eg, severe infections), polycythemia vera, myelofibrosis with myeloid metaplasia. **Decreased in:** Chronic myeloid leukemia, paroxysmal nocturnal hemoglobinuria.	Test may be helpful for distinguishing leukemoid reactions (high-normal or increased LAP) from chronic myeloid leukemia (decreased LAP), but it is poorly reproducible. Ref: Am J Clin Pathol 1963;39:439.
Leukocyte (white blood cell) count, total, Whole blood (WBC count) 3.4–$10 \times 10^3/\mu L$ $[\times 10^9/L]$ ***Panic:*** $< 1.5 \times 10^3/\mu L$ Lavender $	Measure of the total number of leukocytes in whole blood. Counted on automated instruments using light scattering or electrical impedance after lysis of red blood cells. WBCs are distinguished from platelets by size.	**Increased in:** Infection, inflammation, hematologic malignancy, leukemia, lymphoma. Drugs: corticosteroids. **Decreased in:** Aplastic anemia (decreased production), B_{12} or folate deficiency (maturation defect), sepsis (decreased survival). Drugs: phenothiazines, chloramphenicol, aminopyrine.	A spurious increase may be seen when there is a large number of nucleated red cells. Ref: Lab Med 1983;14:509.

	Lipase		
Lipase, serum 0–160 U/L [0–2.66 µkat/L] (laboratory-specific) Marbled $$	Lipases are responsible for hydrolysis of glycerol esters of long-chain fatty acids to produce fatty acids and glycerol. Lipases are produced in the liver, intestine, tongue, stomach, and many other cells. Assays are highly dependent on the substrate used.	**Increased in:** Acute, recurrent, or chronic pancreatitis, pancreatic pseudocyst, pancreatic malignancy, peritonitis, biliary disease, hepatic disease, diabetes mellitus (especially diabetic ketoacidosis), intestinal disease, gastric malignancy or perforation.	The sensitivity of lipase in acute pancreatitis is similar to that of amylase; lipase remains elevated longer than amylase. The specificity of lipase and amylase in acute pancreatitis is similar, though both are poor. Test sensitivity is not very good for chronic pancreatitis or pancreatic cancer. Ref: Arch Pathol Lab Med 1991;115:325. Ref: Clin Chem 1991;37:447. Ref: Dig Dis Sci 1984;29:289.

	Luteinizing hormone		
Luteinizing hormone, serum (LH) Male: 6–30 Female: Premenopause: < 30 Postmenopause: > 35 mIU/mL [IU/L] (laboratory-specific) Marbled $$	LH is stimulated by the hypothalamic hormone gonadotropin-releasing hormone (GnRH). It is secreted from the anterior pituitary and acts on the gonads. LH is the principal regulator of steroid biosynthesis in the ovary and testis.	**Increased in:** Primary hypogonadism, polycystic ovary syndrome, postmenopause. **Decreased in:** Pituitary or hypothalamic failure, anorexia nervosa, severe stress, malnutrition, Kallman's syndrome (gonadotropin deficiency associated with anosmia). Drugs: digoxin, oral contraceptives, phenothiazines.	Intact human chorionic gonadotropin (hCG) cross-reacts with LH in most immunoassays so that LH levels appear to be falsely elevated in pregnancy or in individuals with hCG-secreting tumors. Ref: Clin Obstet Gynecol 1990;33:576.

Test/Range/Collection	Physiologic Basis	Interpretation (sensitivity)	Comments
Lyme disease serology, serum ELISA: negative (< 1:8 titer) Western blot: non-reactive Marbled $$	Test detects the presence of antibody to *Borrelia burgdorferi,* the etiologic agent in Lyme disease, an inflammatory disorder transmitted by the ticks *Ixodes dammini, I pacificus,* and *I scapularis* in the northeastern and midwestern, western, and southeastern USA, respectively. Detects IgM antibody, which develops within 3–6 weeks after the onset of rash; or IgG, which develops within 6–8 weeks after the onset of disease. IgG antibody may persist for months.	**Positive in:** Lyme disease, asymptomatic individuals living in endemic areas, syphilis (*Treponema pallidum*), tick-borne relapsing fever (*Borrelia hermsii*). **Negative:** During the first 5 weeks of infection or after antibiotic therapy.	Test is less sensitive in patients with only a rash. Since culture or direct visualization of the organism is difficult, serologic diagnosis (by ELISA) is indicated, although sensitivity and specificity and standardization of procedure between laboratories need improvement. Cross-reactions may occur with syphilis (should be excluded by RPR and treponemal antibody assays). Ref: Ann Intern Med 1991;114:472. Ref: N Engl J Med 1989;321:586.
Magnesium, serum (Mg²⁺) 1.8–3.0 mg/dL [0.75–1.25 mmol/L] ***Panic:*** < 0.5 or > 4.5 mg/dL Marbled $	Magnesium is primarily an intracellular cation (second most abundant, 60% found in bone); it is a necessary cofactor in numerous enzyme systems, particularly ATPases. In extracellular fluid, it influences neuromuscular response and irritability. Magnesium concentration is determined by intestinal absorption, renal excretion, and exchange with bone and intracellular fluid.	**Increased in:** Dehydration, tissue trauma, renal failure, hypoadrenocorticism, hypothyroidism. Drugs: aspirin (prolonged use), lithium, magnesium salts, progesterone, triamterene. **Decreased in:** Chronic diarrhea, enteric fistula, starvation, chronic alcoholism, total parenteral nutrition with inadequate replacement, hypoparathyroidism (especially post-parathyroid surgery), acute pancreatitis, chronic glomerulonephritis, hyperaldosteronism, diabetic ketoacidosis. Drugs: albuterol, amphotericin B, calcium salts, cisplatin, citrates (blood transfusion), cyclosporine, diuretics, ethacrynic acid.	Hypomagnesemia is associated with tetany, weakness, disorientation, and somnolence. A magnesium deficit may exist with little or no apparent change in serum level. Ref: Arch Intern Med 1988;148:2415.

	MCH	MCHC	MCV
Mean corpuscular hemoglobin, blood (MCH) 26–34 pg Lavender $	The mean corpuscular hemoglobin indicates the amount of hemoglobin per red blood cell in absolute units. A low MCH can mean hypochromia or microcytosis or both. A high MCH is evidence of macrocytosis.	**Increased in:** Macrocytosis. **Decreased in:** Microcytosis (iron deficiency, thalassemia). Hypochromia (lead poisoning, sideroblastic anemia, anemia of chronic disease).	MCH is calculated from measured values of hemoglobin (Hb) and red cell count (RBC) by the formula: $$MCH = Hb / RBC.$$ Ref: Lab Med 1983;14:509. Ref: N Engl J Med 1979;300:1277.
Mean corpuscular hemoglobin concentration, blood (MCHC) 31–36 g/dL [310–360 g/L] Lavender $	MCHC describes how fully the erythrocyte volume is filled with hemoglobin and is calculated from measurement of hemoglobin (Hb), mean corpuscular volume (MCV), and red cell count (RBC) by the formula: $$MCHC = Hb / (MCV \times RBC).$$	**Increased in:** Marked spherocytosis. Spuriously increased in autoagglutination, hemolysis (with spuriously high Hb or low MCV or RBC), lipemia. Cellular dehydration syndromes, xerocytosis. **Decreased in:** Hypochromic anemia (iron deficiency, thalassemia, lead poisoning), sideroblastic anemia, anemia of chronic disease. Spuriously decreased with high white blood cell count, low Hb, or high MCV or RBC.	
Mean corpuscular volume, blood (MCV) 80–100 fL Lavender $	Average volume of the red cell is measured by automated instrument, by electrical impedance, or by light scatter.	**Increased in:** Liver disease, megaloblastic anemia (folate, B_{12} deficiencies), reticulocytosis, newborns. Spurious increase in autoagglutination, high white blood cell count. Drugs: phenytoin. **Decreased in:** Iron deficiency, thalassemia; decreased or normal in anemia of chronic disease.	MCV can be normal in combined iron and folate deficiency. In patients with two red cell populations (macrocytic and microcytic), MCV may be normal. Ref: J Lab Clin Med 1932;17:899.

Test/Range/Collection	Physiologic Basis	Interpretation (sensitivity)	Comments
		Metanephrines	**Methanol**
Metanephrines, urine 0.3–0.9 mg/24 h [1.6–4.9 µmol/d] Urine bottle containing hydrochloric acid $$$ Collect 24-hour urine.	Catecholamines, secreted in excess by pheochromocytomas, are metabolized to metanephrines, and these are excreted in the urine.	**Increased in:** Pheochromocytoma (96%, 98% specificity), neuroblastoma, ganglioneuroma. Drugs: monoamine oxidase inhibitors.	First-line test for diagnosis of pheochromocytoma (see Pheochromocytoma algorithm, p 256). Since < 0.1% of hypertensives have a pheochromocytoma, routine screening of all hypertensives would yield a positive predictive value of < 10%. Avoid overutilization of tests. Do not order urine vanillylmandelic acid, urine catecholamines, and plasma catecholamines at the same time. Plasma catecholamine levels are often spuriously increased when drawn in the hospital setting. Ref: Mayo Clin Proc 1990;65:88.
Methanol, whole blood Negative Green or lavender $$	Serum methanol levels > 20 mg/dL are toxic and levels > 40 mg/dL are life-threatening.	**Increased in:** Methanol intoxication.	Methanol intoxication is associated with metabolic acidosis and an osmolar gap (see Osmolal gap in toxicology, p 267). Methanol is commonly ingested in its pure form or in cleaning and copier solutions. Acute ingestion causes an optic neuritis that may result in blindness. Ref: Med Toxicol 1986;1:309.

Methemoglobin	Metyrapone test
Methemoglobin, whole blood (MetHb) < 0.005 g/dL [< 0.5 g/L] Lavender $$ Analyze promptly.	**Metyrapone test (overnight)**, plasma or serum 8 AM cortisol: < 10 µg/dL [< 280 nmol/L] 8 AM 11-deoxycortisol: > 7 µg/dL [> 202 nmol/L] Marbled, lavender, or green $$$ Give 2.0–2.5 g of metyrapone PO at 12:00 midnight. Draw serum cortisol and 11-deoxycortisol levels at 8:00 AM.
Methemoglobin has its heme iron in the oxidized ferric state and thus cannot combine with and transport oxygen. Methemoglobin can be assayed spectrophotometrically by measuring the decrease in absorbance at 630–635 nm due to the conversion of methemoglobin to cyanmethemoglobin with cyanide.	The metyrapone stimulation test assesses both pituitary and adrenal reserve and is mainly used to diagnose secondary adrenal insufficiency (see Adrenocortical insufficiency algorithm, p. 250). Metyrapone is a drug that inhibits adrenal 11β-hydroxylase and blocks cortisol synthesis. The consequent fall in cortisol increases release of ACTH and hence production of steroids formed proximal to the block (eg, 11-deoxycortisol).
Increased in: Hemoglobin variants (HbM) (rare), methemoglobin reductase deficiency. Oxidant drugs such as sulfonamides (dapsone, sulfasalazine), nitrites and nitrates, aniline dyes, phenacetin.	**Decreased:** An 8 AM 11-deoxycortisol level < 7 µg/dL indicates primary or secondary adrenal insufficiency.
Levels of 1.5 g/dL (10% of total Hb) result in visible cyanosis. Patients with levels of about 35% have headache, weakness, and breathlessness. Levels in excess of 70% are usually fatal. Ref: Am J Med Sci 1985;289:200.	The metyrapone test can be useful in steroid-treated patients to assess the extent of suppression of the pituitary-adrenal axis. Ref: Arch Intern Med 1975;135:698. Ref: JAMA 1979;241:1251.

Test/Range/Collection	Physiologic Basis	Interpretation (sensitivity)	Comments
β₂-Microglobulin, serum (B₂M) < 0.2 mg/dL [< 2.0 mg/L] Marbled $$$	β_2-Microglobulin is a portion of the HLA molecule on cell surfaces and is synthesized by all nucleated cell types and present in all body fluids. It is increased in many conditions that are accompanied by high cell turnover.	**Increased in:** Any type of inflammation, autoimmune disorders, lymphoid malignancies, viral infections (HIV, CMV). Marked elevation in patients with amyloidosis and renal failure.	Of tests used to predict progression to AIDS in HIV-infected patients, CD4 cell number has the most predictive power, followed closely by β_2-microglobulin. Asymptomatic HIV patients with elevated β_2-microglobulin levels have a 2- to 3-fold increased chance of disease progression. Some authors suggest using β_2-microglobulin along with CD4 cells (see p 61) to classify HIV patients and monitor therapy, though no consensus among AIDS experts has been reached. Ref: N Engl J Med 1990;322:166.
Microhemagglutination-*Treponema pallidum* (MHA-TP), serum Nonreactive Marbled $$	The MHA-TP test measures specific antibody against *T pallidum* in a patient's serum by agglutination of *T pallidum* antigen-coated erythrocytes. Antibodies to non-pathogenic treponemes are first removed by binding to nonpathogenic treponemal antigens.	**Increased in:** Syphilis: primary (64–87%), secondary (96–100%), late latent (94–100%), tertiary (94–100%); infectious mononucleosis, collagen-vascular diseases, hyperglobulinemia and dysglobulinemia.	Test is used to confirm reactive serologic tests for syphilis (RPR or VDRL). Compared to FTA-ABS, MHA-TP is slightly less sensitive in all stages of syphilis and becomes reactive somewhat later in the disease. Because test usually remains positive for long periods of time regardless of therapy, it is not useful in assessing the effectiveness of therapy. In a recent study, at 36 months after treatment, 13% had nonreactive MHA-TP tests. Ref: Ann Intern Med 1991;114:1005. Ref: J Infect Dis 1990;162:862. Ref: Ann Intern Med 1986;104:368.

	Neutrophil cytoplasmic antibodies	Oligoclonal bands
Test	**Neutrophil cytoplasmic antibodies,** serum Negative Marbled $$$	**Oligoclonal bands,** serum and CSF Negative Marbled and glass/plastic tube for CSF $$ Collect serum and CSF simultaneously.
Description	Measurement of autoantibodies in serum against cytoplasmic constituents of neutrophils. (See also Autoantibodies table, p 226.)	Electrophoretic examination of IgG in CSF may show oligoclonal bands not found in serum. This suggests local production in CSF of a limited species of IgG.
Positive in	**Positive in:** Wegener's granulomatosis, systemic vasculitis, crescentic glomerulonephritis.	**Positive in:** Multiple sclerosis (88%), CNS syphilis, subacute sclerosing panencephalitis, other CNS inflammatory diseases.
Comment	Test sensitivity for Wegener's granulomatosis ranges from 56% to 96% depending on the population studied. Test specificity for Wegener's granulomatosis is claimed to be high (99%) when requiring diffuse cytoplasmic staining for a positive result, but interpretation is highly technique-dependent. The ability of this assay to reflect disease activity remains unclear. Ref: Ann Intern Med 1989;111:28. Ref: N Engl J Med 1988;318:1651.	Test is indicated only when multiple sclerosis is suspected clinically. Test interpretation is very subjective. IgG index is a more reliable test analytically but neither test is specific for multiple sclerosis. Ref: Mayo Clin Proc 1989;64:577. Ref: Neurology 1985;35:212.

Test/Range/Collection	Physiologic Basis	Interpretation (sensitivity)	Comments
		Osmolality, serum	**Osmolality, urine**
Osmolality, serum (Osm) 285–293 mosm/kg H_2O [mmol/kg H_2O] *Panic:* < 240 or > 320 mosm/kg H_2O Marbled $$	Test measures the osmotic pressure of serum by the freezing point depression method. Plasma and urine osmolality are more useful indicators of degree of hydration than BUN, hematocrit, or serum proteins. Serum osmolality can be estimated by the following formula: $$Osm = 2(Na^+) + \frac{BUN}{2.8} + \frac{glucose}{18}$$	**Increased in:** Diabetic ketoacidosis, nonketotic hyperosmolar hyperglycemic coma, hypernatremia secondary to dehydration (diarrhea, vomiting, fever, hyperventilation, inadequate water intake, central or nephrogenic diabetes insipidus, or osmotic diuresis), hypernatremia with normal hydration (hypothalamic disorders, defective osmostat), hypernatremia with overhydration (iatrogenic or accidental excessive NaCl or $NaHCO_3$ intake), alcohol or other toxic ingestion (see Comments), hypercalcemia; tube feedings. Drugs: corticosteroids, mannitol, glycerin. **Decreased in:** Pregnancy (third trimester), hyponatremia with hypovolemia (adrenal insufficiency, renal losses, diarrhea, vomiting, burns, peritonitis, pancreatitis), hyponatremia with normovolemia (congestive heart failure, cirrhosis, nephrotic syndrome, SIADH, postoperative state). Drugs: chlorthalidone, cyclophosphamide, thiazides.	If the difference between calculated and measured serum osmolality is greater than 10 mosm/kg H_2O, suspect a low-molecular-weight toxin (alcohol, methanol, isopropyl alcohol, ethylene glycol, acetone, ethyl ether, paraldehyde, or mannitol). (See Osmolal gap in toxicology, p 267, for further explanation.) Most commonly, ethanol increases serum osmolality by 22 mosm/kg H_2O for every 100 mg/dL alcohol. A normal serum osmolality excludes ethanol intoxication. Ref: Am J Clin Pathol 1973;60:695. Ref: Am J Med 1982;72:308.
Osmolality, urine (Urine Osm) Random: 100–900 mosm/kg H_2O [mmol/kg H_2O] Urine container $$	Test measures renal tubular concentrating ability.	**Increased in:** Hypovolemia. Drugs: anesthetic agents (during surgery), carbamazepine, chlorpropamide, cyclophosphamide, metolazone, vincristine. **Decreased in:** Diabetes insipidus, primary polydipsia, exercise, starvation. Drugs: acetohexamide, demeclocycline, glyburide, lithium, tolazamide.	With average fluid intake, normal random urine osmolality is 100–900 mosm/kg H_2O. After 12-hour fluid restriction, normal random urine osmolality is > 850 mosm/kg H_2O. Ref: Am J Med 1982;72:308.

		Oxygen
Oxygen, partial pressure, whole blood (PO_2) 83–108 mm Hg [11.04–14.36 kPa] Heparinized syringe $$$ Collect arterial blood in a heparinized syringe. Send to laboratory immediately on ice.	Test measures the partial pressure of oxygen (oxygen tension) in arterial blood. Partial pressure of oxygen is critical since it determines (along with hemoglobin and blood supply) tissue oxygen supply.	**Increased in:** Oxygen therapy. **Decreased in:** Ventilation/perfusion mismatching (asthma, COPD, atelectasis, pulmonary embolism, pneumonia, interstitial lung disease, airway obstruction by foreign body, shock); alveolar hypoventilation (kyphoscoliosis, neuromuscular disease, head injury, stroke); right-to-left shunt (congenital heart disease). Drugs: barbiturates, narcotics.	% saturation of hemoglobin (SO_2) represents the oxygen content divided by the oxygen carrying capacity of hemoglobin. % saturation on blood gas reports is calculated not measured. It is calculated from PO_2 and pH using reference oxyhemoglobin dissociation curves for normal adult hemoglobin (lacking methemoglobin, carboxyhemoglobin, etc). At $PO_2 < 60$ mm Hg, the oxygen saturation (and content) cannot be reliably estimated from the PO_2. Therefore, oximetry should be used to determine % saturation directly. Ref: JAMA 1990;264:244.

	Parathyroid hormone	
Test/Range/Collection	**Physiologic Basis**	**Interpretation (sensitivity)**	**Comments**

Test/Range/Collection	Physiologic Basis	Interpretation (sensitivity)	Comments
Parathyroid hormone (PTH), serum Intact PTH: 11–54 pg/mL [1.2–5.7 pmol/L] (laboratory-specific) Marbled $$$$ Fasting sample preferred; simultaneous measurement of serum calcium and phosphorus is also required.	PTH is secreted from the parathyroid glands. It mobilizes calcium from bone, increases distal renal tubular reabsorption of calcium, decreases proximal renal tubular reabsorption of phosphorus, and stimulates 1,25-hydroxy vitamin D synthesis from 25-hydroxy vitamin D by renal 1α-hydroxylase. The "intact" PTH molecule (84 amino acids) has a circulating half-life of about 5 minutes. Carboxy-terminal and midmolecule fragments make up 90% of circulating PTH. They are biologically inactive, cleared by the kidney, and have half-lives of about 1–2 hours. The amino-terminal fragment is biologically active and has a half-life of about 1–2 minutes. Measurement of PTH by immunoassay depends on the specificity of the antibodies used.	**Increased in:** Primary hyperparathyroidism, secondary hyperparathyroidism due to renal disease. Drugs: lithium, furosemide, phosphates. **Decreased in:** Hypoparathyroidism, sarcoidosis, hyperthyroidism, hypomagnesemia, malignancy with hypercalcemia, nonparathyroid hypercalcemia.	PTH results must always be evaluated in light of concurrent serum calcium levels (see PTH and calcium nomogram, p 268). PTH tests differ in sensitivity and specificity from assay to assay and from laboratory to laboratory. C-terminal antibody measures intact, carboxy-terminal and midmolecule fragments. It is 85% sensitive and 95% specific for primary hyperparathyroidism. N-terminal antibody measures intact and amino-terminal fragments. It is about 75% sensitive for hyperparathyroidism. Intact PTH assays are preferred because they detect PTH suppression in nonparathyroid hypercalcemia. Ref: Endocrinol Metab Clin North Am 1989;18:647. Ref: Ann Intern Med 1987;106:559. Ref: Arch Surg 1986;121:841.

PTT	pH
Partial thromboplastin time, activated, plasma (PTT) 25–35 seconds (range varies) *Panic:* ≥ 60 seconds Blue $$ Fill tube adequately. Do not contaminate specimen with heparin.	**pH**, whole blood Arterial: 7.35–7.45 Venous: 7.31–7.41 Heparinized syringe $$$ Specimen must be collected in heparinized syringe and immediately transported on ice to lab without exposure to air.
Patient's plasma is activated to clot in vitro by mixing it with phospholipid and an activator substance. Test screens the intrinsic coagulation pathway and adequacy of all coagulation factors except XIII and VII. PTT is usually abnormal if any factor level drops below 30–40% of normal.	pH assesses the acid-base status of blood, an extremely useful measure of integrated cardiorespiratory function. The essential relationship between pH, PCO_2 and bicarbonate (HCO_3^-) is expressed by the Henderson–Hasselbalch equation (at 37 °C): $$pH = 6.1 + \log\left(\frac{HCO_3^-}{PCO_2 \times 0.03}\right)$$ Arteriovenous pH difference is 0.01–0.03 but is greater in patients with congestive heart failure and shock.
Increased in: Deficiency of any individual coagulation factor except XIII and VII, specific factor inhibitors (eg, lupus anticoagulant), nonspecific inhibitors (eg, von Willebrand's disease (PTT may also be normal), hemophilia A and B, disseminated intravascular coagulation (DIC). Drugs: heparin, warfarin. **Decreased in:** Hypercoagulable states, DIC.	**Increased in:** *Respiratory alkalosis:* hyperventilation (eg, anxiety), sepsis, liver disease, fever, early salicylate poisoning, and excessive artificial ventilation. *Metabolic alkalosis:* Loss of gastric HCl (eg, vomiting), potassium depletion, excessive alkali administration (eg, bicarbonate, antacids), diuretics, volume depletion. **Decreased in:** *Respiratory acidosis:* decreased alveolar ventilation (eg, COPD, respiratory depressants), neuromuscular diseases (eg, myasthenia). *Metabolic acidosis* (bicarbonate deficit): increased formation of acids (eg, ketoacidosis); increased H^+ excretion (eg, renal failure, renal tubular acidosis, Fanconi's syndrome); increased acid intake (eg, ion-exchange resins, salicylates, ammonium chloride, ethylene glycol, methanol); and increased loss of alkaline body fluids (eg, diarrhea, fistulas, aspiration of gastrointestinal contents, biliary drainage).
PTT is the best test to monitor adequacy of heparin therapy. Test is not always abnormal in von Willebrand's disease. Test may be normal in chronic DIC. A very common cause of PTT prolongation is the spurious presence of heparin in the plasma sample. Ref: JAMA 1989;262:2428.	The pH of a standing sample decreases because of cellular metabolism. The correction of pH (measured at 37 °C), based on the patient's temperature, is not clinically useful. (See also Acid-base nomogram, p 261.) Ref: Am J Med 1982;72:496.

Test/Range/Collection	Physiologic Basis	Interpretation (sensitivity)	Comments
Phosphorus, serum 2.5–4.5 mg/dL [0.8–1.45 mmol/L] *Panic:* < 1.0 mg/dL Marbled $ Avoid hemolysis.	The plasma concentration of inorganic phosphate is determined by parathyroid gland function, action of vitamin D, intestinal absorption, renal function, bone metabolism, and nutrition.	**Increased in:** Renal failure, massive blood transfusion, hypoparathyroidism, sarcoidosis, neoplasms, adrenal insufficiency, acromegaly, hypervitaminosis D, osteolytic metastases to bone, leukemia, milk-alkali syndrome, healing bone fractures, pseudohypoparathyroidism, diabetes mellitus with ketosis, malignant hyperpyrexia, cirrhosis, lactic acidosis, respiratory acidosis. Drugs: phosphate infusions or enemas, anabolic steroids, ergocalciferol, furosemide, hydrochlorothiazide, and others. **Decreased in:** Hyperparathyroidism, hypovitaminosis D (rickets, osteomalacia), malabsorption (steatorrhea), malnutrition, starvation or cachexia, GH deficiency, chronic alcoholism, severe diarrhea, vomiting, nasogastric suction, severe burns (diuretic phase), acute gout, osteoblastic metastases to bone, inadequate phosphate repletion, carbohydrate administration (intravenous), renal tubular acidosis and other renal tubular defects, diabetic ketoacidosis (during recovery), acid-base disturbances, hypokalemia, pregnancy, hypothyroidism. Drugs: phosphate-binding antacids, anticonvulsants, estrogens, isoniazid, oral contraceptives, prolonged use of thiazides, glucose infusion, salicylates (toxicity).	Ref: N Engl J Med 1985;313:447.

Phosphorus

	Platelet aggregation	Platelet count
Test / Specimen	**Platelet aggregation, whole blood** Aggregation by adenosine diphosphate (ADP), collagen, epinephrine, thrombin, ristocetin, and arachidonic acid Drawn by lab $$$$ Whole blood in citrate is drawn into a plastic tube. Platelet-rich plasma (PRP) is obtained by centrifuging at $100 \times g$ for 10–15 minutes.	**Platelet count, whole blood (Plt)** $150–450 \times 10^3/\mu L$ $[\times 10^9/L]$ **Panic:** $< 25 \times 10^3/\mu L$ Lavender $
Description	Platelet aggregometry can provide information concerning possible qualitative platelet defects. Aggregation is measured as an increase in light transmission through stirred PRP when a specific agonist is added. Test examines platelet aggregation response to various agonists (eg, ADP, collagen, epinephrine, thrombin, ristocetin).	Platelets are released from megakaryocytes in bone marrow and are important for normal hemostasis. Platelet counting is done by a flow cytometry based on size discrimination using either electrical impedance or electro-optical systems.
Interpretation	**Abnormal in:** Acquired defects in the platelet release reaction (eg, drugs, following cardiopulmonary bypass, uremia), congenital release abnormalities, Glanzmann's thrombasthenia (absent aggregation to ADP, collagen, epinephrine), storage pool disease (no secondary wave with ADP, epinephrine, and decreased aggregation with collagen), and von Willebrand's disease (normal aggregation with all factors except ristocetin). Drugs: aspirin.	**Increased in:** Myeloproliferative disorders: polycythemia vera, chronic myeloid leukemia, essential thrombocythemia, myelofibrosis; after bleeding, postsplenectomy, reactive thrombocytosis secondary to inflammatory diseases, iron deficiency, alkalosis. **Decreased in:** Decreased production: bone marrow suppression or replacement, chemotherapeutic agents, drugs (eg, ethanol). Increased destruction or removal: splenomegaly, disseminated intravascular coagulation, platelet antibodies (idiopathic thrombocytopenic purpura, posttransfusion purpura, neonatal isoimmune thrombocytopenia, drugs [eg, quinidine, cephalosporins]).
Comments / Reference	Test should not be done if the patient has taken aspirin within the previous 10 days. Direct PRP aggregation by ristocetin (1.5 mg/mL) may be normal or abnormal in von Willebrand's disease (vWD). Because this test has limited sensitivity to detect vWD, it is no longer used to diagnose vWD (see instead Bleeding time, p 54, and von Willebrand factor protein, p 142). Ref: N Engl J Med 1991;324:27.	Ref: Am J Clin Pathol 1965;44:678. Ref: Med Lab Sci 1976;33:201.

Test/Range/Collection	Physiologic Basis	Interpretation (sensitivity)	Comments
Platelet-associated IgG, whole blood Negative Yellow $$$$ 17 mL of blood is needed.	Antibody screening involves direct testing of a patient's platelets to demonstrate platelet-associated IgG (which may be directed against specific platelet antigens or which may represent immune complexes nonspecifically absorbed to the platelet surface) in idiopathic (autoimmune) thrombocytopenic purpura (ITP). It also involves indirect testing of the patient's serum against a panel of reagent platelets to detect circulating antiplatelet antibodies. In alloimmune thrombocytopenia, the patient's direct test is negative and the patient's serum reacts with reagent platelets. Antibody specificity can be identified, and platelets lacking the involved antigen can be transfused.	**Positive in:** Some autoimmune thrombocytopenias (eg, ITP) (90–95%).	In ITP, the direct antiplatelet antibody test may be useful to confirm the diagnosis and monitor subsequent response to therapy. It is also useful in diagnosing posttransfusion purpura and suspected neonatal isoimmune thrombocytopenia. Platelet-associated IgG is also a diagnostic test for patients with thrombocytopenia or as part of a platelet crossmatch prior to transfusion of patients who have repeatedly failed to respond to random donor platelet transfusions. Ref: Rose NR et al (editors): *Manual of Clinical Laboratory Immunology.* American Society for Microbiology, 1986.
Porphobilinogen, urine (PBG) Negative $$ Protect from light.	Porphyrias are characterized clinically by neurologic and cutaneous manifestations and chemically by overproduction of porphyrin and other precursors of heme production. PBG is a water-soluble precursor of heme whose urinary excretion is increased in symptomatic hepatic porphyrias.	**Positive in:** Acute intermittent porphyria, variegate porphyria, coproporphyria, lead poisoning (rare). **Negative in:** 20–30% of patients with hepatic porphyria between attacks.	Positive qualitative urinary PBG tests should be followed up by quantitative measurements. Specific porphyrias can be better defined by quantitative measurement of urine PBG and by measurement of erythrocyte uroporphyrinogen-1-synthetase. A screening PBG test is insensitive and a negative test does not rule out a diagnosis of porphyria, especially the carrier state. Ref: Am J Clin Pathol 1989;92:644. Ref: Mayo Clin Proc 1982;57:454.

	Potassium	Prolactin
Potassium, serum (K^+) 3.5–5.0 meq/L [mmol/L] ***Panic:*** < 3.0 or > 6.0 meq/L Marbled $ Avoid hemolysis.	Potassium is predominantly an intracellular cation whose plasma level is regulated by renal excretion. Plasma potassium concentration determines neuromuscular irritability. Elevated or depressed potassium concentrations interfere with muscle contraction.	Prolactin is a polypeptide hormone secreted by the anterior pituitary. It functions in the initiation and maintenance of lactation in the postpartum period. PRL secretion is inhibited by hypothalamic secretion of dopamine. Prolactin levels increase with renal failure, hypothyroidism, and drugs that are dopamine antagonists.
	Increased in: Massive hemolysis, severe tissue damage, rhabdomyolysis, acidosis, dehydration, acute or chronic renal failure, Addison's disease, renal tubular acidosis type IV (hyporeninemic hypoaldosteronism), hyperkalemic familial periodic paralysis. Drugs: potassium salts, potassium-sparing diuretics (eg, spironolactone, triamterene), nonsteroidal anti-inflammatory drugs, beta-blockers, ACE inhibitors. **Decreased in:** Low potassium intake, prolonged vomiting or diarrhea, renal tubular acidosis types I and II, hyperaldosteronism, Cushing's syndrome, osmotic diuresis (eg, hyperglycemia), alkalosis, familial periodic paralysis. Drugs: diuretics.	**Increased in:** Sleep, nursing, nipple stimulation, exercise, hypoglycemia, stress, hypothyroidism, pituitary tumors (prolactinomas and others), hypothalamic/pituitary stalk lesions, renal failure. Drugs: phenothiazines, haloperidol, reserpine, methyldopa, estrogens, opiates, cimetidine. **Decreased in:** Drugs: levodopa.
	Spurious hyperkalemia can occur with hemolysis of sample, delayed separation of serum from erythrocytes, prolonged fist clenching during blood drawing, prolonged tourniquet placement, and very high white blood cell or platelet counts. For severe hyperkalemia, first give calcium to stabilize heart muscle cells and then give glucose and insulin. Ref: J Gen Intern Med 1986;1:368.	Serum PRL is used primarily in workup of suspected pituitary tumor (60% of pituitary adenomas secrete PRL). Clinical presentation is usually amenorrhea and galactorrhea in women and impotence in men. (See Amenorrhea algorithm, p 251.) Only 4% of impotence is caused by hyperprolactinemia, and hyperprolactinemia is rare in the absence of low serum testosterone. Ref: Lancet 1982;2:129.

Test/Range/Collection	Physiologic Basis	Interpretation (sensitivity)	Comments
Prostate-specific antigen, serum (PSA) 0–4 ng/mL [µg/L] Marbled $$$	Prostate-specific antigen is a glyco-protein produced by cells of the prostatic ductal epithelium and is present in the serum of all men. It is absent from the serum of women.	**Increased in:** Prostate carcinoma, benign prostatic hypertrophy (BPH), following prostate examination. **Negative in:** Metastatic prostate carcinoma treated with antiandrogen therapy, postprostatectomy.	PSA is used to monitor recurrence of treated prostate cancer. Use of PSA for cancer screening is controversial because PSA is often increased in BPH and there is low predictive value of a positive test when performed in healthy older men. PSA replaces the acid phosphatase test. Ref: N Engl J Med 1987;317:909. Ref: N Engl J Med 1991;324:1156.
Protein C, plasma 71–176% Blue $$$	Test measures activity of protein C, a vitamin K-dependent proenzyme synthesized in the liver. It exerts an anticoagulant effect through inactivation of factors Va and VIIIc after it is activated by thrombin. Protein C is inactive unless protein S is available as cofactor. Deficiency is inherited in an auto-somal-dominant fashion with incomplete penetrance.	**Decreased in:** Congenital deficiency, liver disease, cirrhosis (13–25%), warfarin use (28–60%), vitamin K deficiency, disseminated intravascular coagulation (DIC).	Homozygous deficiency of protein C (< 1% activity) is associated with fatal neonatal purpura fulminans and massive venous thrombosis. Heterozygous patients (1 in 200–300 of the population, with levels 25–50% of normal) may be at risk for venous thrombosis. Interpretation of an abnormally low protein C must be tempered by the clinical setting. Anticoagulant therapy, DIC, and liver disease must not be present. There is overlap between lower limits of normal values and values found in heterozygotes. Ref: N Engl J Med 1986;314:1298. Ref: Semin Thromb Hemost 1984; 10:162.

	Protein electrophoresis	Protein S

Protein electrophoresis, serum

Adults:
Albumin: 3.3–5.7
α_1: 0.1–0.4
α_2: 0.3–0.9
β: 0.7–1.5
γ: 0.5–1.4 g/dL

Marbled
$$

Electrophoresis of serum will separate serum proteins into albumin, α_1, α_2, β_2, and γ fractions. Albumin is the principal serum protein (see Albumin, p 44). The α_1 fraction contains α_1-antitrypsin and α_1-acid glycoprotein. The α_2 fraction contains α_2-macroglobulin, haptoglobin, and ceruloplasmin. The β fraction contains transferrin, hemopexin, complement C3, and β-lipoproteins. The γ fraction contains immunoglobulins G, A, D, E, and M.

↑α_1: inflammatory states (α_1-antitrypsin is an acute phase reactant).
↑α_2: nephrotic syndrome, inflammatory states, oral contraceptives.
↑β: hyperlipidemia, hemoglobinemia secondary to hemolysis.
↑γ: polyclonal gammopathies (liver disease, cirrhosis [associated with β-γ "bridging"], chronic infections, autoimmune disease); monoclonal gammopathies (multiple myeloma, Waldenström's macroglobulinemia, lymphoid malignancies, monoclonal gammopathy of uncertain significance).
↓α_1: hereditary α_1-antitrypsin deficiency.
↓α_2: in vivo hemolysis.
↓β: hypo-β-lipoproteinemias.
↓γ: immune deficiency.

Presence of "spikes" in α_2, β_2, or γ regions necessitates the use of immunoelectrophoresis to verify the presence of a monoclonal gammopathy (see Immunoelectrophoresis, p 96).
If Bence Jones proteins (light chains) are suspected, urine protein electrophoresis needs to be done.
Test is insensitive for detection of decreased levels of immunoglobulins and α_1-antitrypsin. Specific quantitation is required (see Immunoglobulins, p 96, and α_1-Antitrypsin, p 53).
If plasma is used, fibrinogen will be detected in the β-γ region.
Ref: Mayo Clin Proc 1978;53:719.

Protein S (antigen), plasma

76–178%

Blue
$$$

Protein S is a vitamin K-dependent glycoprotein, synthesized in the liver.
It acts as a cofactor for protein C in producing its anticoagulant effect. 60% of protein S is protein-bound; only free protein S has anticoagulant function.
Deficiency is associated with recurrent venous thrombosis before the age of 40.

Decreased in: Congenital protein S deficiency, liver disease, warfarin therapy, disseminated intravascular coagulation, vitamin K deficiency, nephrotic syndrome.

Protein S is measured by enzyme immunoassay. This measures antigen and not biologic activity.
Protein S can also be measured in a functional assay.
Ref: Ann Intern Med 1985;102:814.
Ref: Ann Intern Med 1987;106:677.

Test/Range/Collection	Physiologic Basis	Interpretation (sensitivity)	Comments
Protein, total, plasma or serum 6.0–8.0 g/dL [60–80 g/L] Marbled $ Avoid prolonged venous stasis during collection.	The plasma protein concentration is determined by the nutritional state, hepatic function, renal function, hydration, and various disease states. The plasma protein concentration determines the colloidal osmotic pressure.	**Increased in:** Polyclonal or monoclonal gammopathies, marked dehydration. Drugs: anabolic steroids, androgens, corticosteroids, epinephrine. **Decreased in:** Protein-losing enteropathies, acute burns, nephrotic syndrome, severe dietary protein deficiency, chronic liver disease, malabsorption syndrome, agammaglobulinemia.	The serum total protein consists primarily of albumin and globulin. Hypoproteinemia usually means hypoalbuminemia, since albumin is the major serum protein. The serum globulin level is calculated as total protein minus albumin.
Prothrombin time, whole blood (PT) 11–15 seconds ***Panic:*** ≥ 30 seconds Blue $ Fill tube completely.	PT screens the extrinsic pathway of the coagulation system. It is performed by adding calcium and tissue thromboplastin to a sample of citrated, platelet-poor plasma and measuring the time required for fibrin clot formation. It is most sensitive to deficiencies in the vitamin K–dependent clotting factors II, VII, IX, and X. It is also sensitive to deficiencies of factor V. It is insensitive to fibrinogen deficiency and not affected by heparin. PT is also used to monitor warfarin therapy.	**Increased in:** Liver disease, vitamin K deficiency, intravascular coagulation, circulating anticoagulant, massive transfusion. Drugs: warfarin.	In liver disease, the PT reflects the hepatic capacity for protein synthesis. PT responds rapidly to altered hepatic function because the serum half-lives of factors II and VII are short (hours). Routine preoperative measurement of PT is unnecessary unless there is a clinical history of a bleeding disorder. Efforts to standardize and report the prothrombin time as an INR (International Normalized Ratio) depend on assigning reagents an International Sensitivity Index (ISI) so that INR = $$\left(\dfrac{PT_{Patient}}{PT_{Normal}}\right)^{ISI}$$ However, assignment of incorrect ISI by reagent manufacturers has caused a greater lack of standardization. Ref: Arch Surg 1982;117:48. Ref: JAMA 1989;262:2428.

	Physiologic Basis	Increased in	Comments
Q Fever antibody, serum <1:8 titer Marbled $$$ Submit paired sera, one collected within 1 week of illness and another 2–3 weeks later. Avoid hemolysis.	*Coxiella burnetii* is a rickettsial organism that is the causative organism for Q fever. Antibodies produced in response to the organism can be detected by the presence of agglutinins or by complement fixation (CF). Agglutinin titers are found 5–8 days after infection. CF antibodies can be seen at 2 weeks. A 4-fold rise in titer is considered diagnostic.	**Increased in:** Acute or chronic Q fever (CF antibodies are present by the second week in 65% of cases and by the fourth week in 90%), and recent vaccination for Q fever.	Occasionally, titers do not rise for 4–6 weeks, especially if antimicrobial therapy has been given. Recent Q fever vaccination will cause a rise equal to that seen with acute infection. Antibodies for Q fever do not cross-react with other rickettsial antibodies. Ref: Rev Inf Dis 1987;9:935.
Rapid plasma reagin, serum (RPR) Nonreactive Marbled $	Measures nontreponemal antibodies that are produced when *Treponema pallidum* interacts with host tissue. The card test is a flocculation test performed by using a cardiolipin-lecithin-cholesterol carbon-containing antigen mixed on a card with the patient's serum. A positive test (presence of antibodies) is indicated when black carbon clumps produced by flocculation are seen by the naked eye.	**Increased in:** Syphilis: primary (78%), secondary (97%), symptomatic late (74%). Biologic false-positives occur in a wide variety of conditions, including leprosy, malaria, intravenous drug abuse, aging, infectious mononucleosis, autoimmune diseases (SLE, rheumatoid arthritis), pregnancy.	RPR is used as a screening test and in suspected primary and secondary syphilis. Since the test lacks specificity, positive tests should be confirmed with the FTA-ABS or MHA-TP test (see p 80 and p 108, respectively). RPR titers can be used to follow serologic response to treatment. (See Syphilis test table, p 240.) In a recent study, 72% of patients with initial episodes of primary syphilis and 56% with initial episodes of secondary syphilis had seroreverted the RPR test result within 36 months. Patients with their first syphilis infection are more likely to serorevert than those with repeated infections. The RPR reversal rate also depends on the pretreatment titer and the stage of the disease. Ref: Ann Intern Med 1991;114:1005. Ref: Ann Intern Med 1986;104:368.

Test/Range/Collection	Physiologic Basis	Interpretation (sensitivity)	Comments
	Red cell volume		**Renin activity**
Red cell volume, whole blood (RCV) Male: 24–32 Female: 22–28 mL/kg Yellow Lavender (for Hct) $$$	Test measures absolute volume of red cells based on hemodilution of a known quantity of radioactivity in the circulation. Test can distinguish between absolute polycythemia (increased hematocrit [Hct], increased RCV) and relative polycythemia (hemoconcentration) (increased Hct, normal RCV). A sample of the patient's whole blood is labeled with radioactive ^{51}Cr (which is taken up into red cells) and reinjected into the patient. Blood is sampled 10 and 60 minutes later to measure radioactivity.	**Increased in:** Polycythemia vera, secondary polycythemia due to tissue hypoxemia (pulmonary disease, congenital heart disease, carboxyhemoglobinemia [cigarette smoking], methemoglobinemia), or neoplasms (renal cell carcinoma, hepatoma, large uterine leiomyomas), high altitude, pregnancy.	Test is clinically indicated in the diagnosis of polycythemia vera. Ref: J Nucl Med 1980;21:793. Ref: Semin Nucl Med 1975;5:63.
Renin activity, plasma (PRA) *High-sodium diet* (75–150 meq Na⁺/d): supine: 0.2–2.3 standing: 1.3–4.0 ng/mL/h *Low-sodium diet* (30–75 meq Na⁺/d): standing: 4.0–7.7 ng/mL/h Lavender $$	The renal juxtaglomerular apparatus generates renin, an enzyme that converts angiotensinogen to angiotensin I. The inactive angiotensin I is then converted to angiotensin II, which is a potent vasopressor. Renin activity is measured by the ability of patient's plasma to generate angiotensin I from substrate (angiotensinogen). Normal values depend on the patient's hydration, posture, and salt intake.	**Increased in:** Dehydration, some hypertensive states (eg, renal artery stenosis); edematous states (cirrhosis, nephrotic syndrome, congestive heart failure); hypokalemic states (gastrointestinal sodium and potassium loss, Bartter's syndrome); adrenal insufficiency. Drugs: ACE inhibitors, estrogen, hydralazine, nifedipine, minoxidil, oral contraceptives. **Decreased in:** Hyporeninemic hypoaldosteronism, some hypertensive states (eg, primary aldosteronism). Drugs: beta-blockers, aspirin, clonidine, prazosin, reserpine, methyldopa, indomethacin.	PRA alone is not a satisfactory screening tests for hyperaldosteronism because suppressed PRA has only 64% sensitivity and 83% specificity for primary hyperaldosteronism. However, when plasma aldosterone and PRA testing are combined, the sensitivity for primary hyperaldosteronism increases to 95% (see Aldosterone, plasma, p 44). Test is also useful in evaluation of hypoaldosteronism (low-sodium diet, patient standing). Measurement of peripheral vein renin activity is not useful in classification of hypertensive patients. Bilateral renal vein sampling has been used to investigate renal artery stenosis. Ref: Am J Med 1983;74:641.

Reptilase clotting time	Reticulocyte count	Rh grouping
When the thrombin time is prolonged, the reptilase time is useful in distinguishing the presence of an antithrombin (normal reptilase time) from hypo- or dysfibrinogenemia (prolonged reptilase time). The reptilase time is normal when heparin is the cause of a prolonged thrombin time. The reptilase time is only slightly prolonged by fibrin degradation products. Ref: Br J Haematol 1971;21:43.	This test is indicated in the evaluation of anemia to distinguish hypoproliferative from hemolytic anemia or blood loss. The old method of measuring reticulocytes (manual staining and counting) has poor reproducibility. It has been replaced by fluorescence-activated flow cytometry. Ref: Lab Med 1989;20:551.	Ref: *Technical Manual of the American Association of Blood Banks*, 10th ed. American Association of Blood Banks, 1990.
Increased in: Hypo-, dys-, and afibrinogenemia. **Normal in:** Presence of heparin.	**Increased in:** Hemolytic anemia, blood loss; recovery from iron, B_{12}, or folate deficiency or drug-induced anemia. **Decreased in:** Iron deficiency anemia, aplastic anemia, anemia of chronic disease, megaloblastic anemia, sideroblastic anemia, bone marrow suppression, autoimmune hemolytic anemias.	
Reptilase is an enzyme derived from the venom of *Bothrops atrox* or *Bothrops jararaca*, South American pit vipers. Reptilase cleaves a fibrinopeptide from fibrinogen directly, bypassing the heparin-antithrombin system, and produces a fibrin clot. The reptilase time will be normal in heparin toxicity, even when the thrombin time is infinite.	Reticulocytes are immature red blood cells that contain cytoplasmic mRNA.	The terms Rh (Rhesus) positive and negative refer to the presence or absence of the red cell antigen, D. It is, after A and B, the next most important red cell antigen in transfusion practice. Persons whose red cells lack D do not regularly have anti-D in their serum. Formation of anti-D almost always results from exposure through transfusion or pregnancy to red cells possessing the D antigen. Of D– persons receiving a single D+ unit, 50–75% will develop anti-D. The blood of all donors and recipients is therefore routinely tested for D, so that D– recipients can be given D– blood. Donor bloods must also be tested for a weak form of D antigen, called D^u and be labeled D+, if the D^u test is positive. Recipient blood need not be tested for D^u.
Reptilase clotting time, plasma 13–19 seconds Blue $$	**Reticulocyte count,** whole blood $33\text{–}137 \times 10^3/\mu L$ $[\times 10^9/L]$ Lavender $	**Rh grouping,** red cells (Rh) Red or lavender $ Proper identification of specimen is critical.

Test/Range/Collection	Physiologic Basis	Interpretation (sensitivity)	Comments
Rheumatoid factor, serum (RF) Negative (< 1:16) Marbled $	Heterogeneous autoantibodies usually of the IgM class that react against the Fc region of human IgG.	**Positive in:** Rheumatoid arthritis (75–90%), Sjögren's syndrome (80–90%), scleroderma, dermatomyositis, SLE (30%), sarcoidosis, Waldenström's macroglobulinemia. Drugs: methyldopa, others. Low titer RF can be found in healthy older patients (20%), 1–4% of normal individuals, and in a variety of acute immune responses (eg, viral infections, infectious mononucleosis, and viral hepatitis), chronic infections (tuberculosis, leprosy, subacute infective endocarditis), and chronic active hepatitis.	Rheumatoid factor can be useful in differentiating rheumatoid arthritis from other chronic inflammatory arthritides. However, a positive RF test is only one of several criteria needed to make the diagnosis of rheumatoid arthritis. (See also Autoantibodies table, p 226). Ref: Geriatrics 1989;44:61.
Rubella antibody, serum < 1:8 titer Marbled $ For diagnosis of a recent infection, submit paired sera, one collected within 1 week of illness and another 2–3 weeks later.	Rubella (German measles) is a viral infection that causes fever, malaise, coryza, lymphadenopathy, fine maculopapular rash, and congenital birth defects when the fetus is infected in utero. Antibodies to rubella can be detected by hemagglutination inhibition (HI), complement fixation (CF), or solid phase immunoassay techniques. Titers usually appear as rash fades (1 week) and peak at 10–14 days for HI and 4–8 weeks for CF. Baseline titers may remain elevated for life.	**Increased in:** Recent rubella infection, congenital rubella infection, previous rubella infection or vaccination (immunity). Spuriously increased IgM antibody occurs in the presence of rheumatoid factor.	Rubella antibody titers of ≤ 1:8 indicate lack of immunity. Titers of > 1:32 indicate immunity from prior infection or vaccination. Definitive diagnosis of acute infections is based on a 4-fold rise in titer or presence of IgM antibody. To diagnose congenital infection, submit a single specimen. If positive, submit second specimen 2–3 months later to rule out maternal antibody transmission across the placenta. Ref: Rev Infect Dis 1985;7:S108.

		Russell's viper venom clotting time	Salicylate
Russell's viper venom clotting time (dilute), plasma (RVVT) 24–37 seconds Blue $$	Russell viper venom is extracted from a pit viper (*Vipera russelli*), which is common in Southeast Asia (especially Burma) and which causes a rapidly fatal syndrome of consumptive coagulopathy with hemorrhage, shock, rhabdomyolysis, and renal failure. Approximately 70% of the protein content of the venom is phospholipase A_2, which activates factor X in the presence of phospholipid, bypassing factor VII. RVVT is a phospholipid-dependent coagulation test. It is used in detection of antiphospholipid antibodies (so-called lupus anticoagulants). It should be noted that the anticoagulant detected in vitro may be associated with thrombosis (and not bleeding) in vivo.	**Increased in:** Circulating lupus anticoagulants, severe fibrinogen deficiency (< 50 mg/dL), deficiencies in prothrombin, factor V, factor X, and heparin therapy. **Normal in:** Factor VII deficiency and all intrinsic pathway factor deficiencies.	The lupus anticoagulant may be associated with a prolonged PTT and a positive inhibitor screen (mixing study). If heparin is not present, a diluted Russell viper venom test may be indicated to confirm that the inhibitor is a lupus anticoagulant. Since specific factor inhibitors against factors VIII and IX are associated with clinically significant bleeding and require specific treatment, they must not be missed. The lupus anticoagulant is associated with an increased risk of thrombosis (venous > arterial), recurrent spontaneous abortion, and the primary antiphospholipid syndrome of arterial thrombosis. Ref: Haemostasis 1990;20:208. Ref: Prog Hemost 1982;6:263.
Salicylate, serum (Aspirin) 20–30 mg/dL [200–300 mg/L] ***Panic:*** > 35 mg/dL Marbled $$	At high concentrations, salicylate stimulates hyperventilation, uncouples oxidative phosphorylation, and impairs glucose and fatty acid metabolism. Salicylate toxicity is thus marked by respiratory alkalosis and metabolic acidosis.	**Increased in:** Acute or chronic salicylate intoxication.	The potential toxicity of salicylate levels after acute ingestion can be determined by using the Salicylate nomogram, p. 272. Nomograms have become less valid with the increasing popularity of enteric-coated slow-release aspirin preparations. Critical level is > 35 mg/dL. Ref: Pediatrics 1960;26:800.

Test/Range/Collection	Physiologic Basis	Interpretation (sensitivity)	Comments
Semen analysis, ejaculate Sperm count: $> 20 \times 10^6$/mL [10^9/L] Motility score: $> 60\%$ motile Volume: 2–5 mL Normal morphology: $> 60\%$ $$ Semen is collected in a urine container after masturbation following 3 days of abstinence from ejaculation. Specimen must be examined promptly.	Sperm is viewed under the microscope for motility and morphology. Infertility can be associated with low counts or with sperm of abnormal morphology or decreased motility.	**Decreased in:** Primary or secondary testicular failure, cryptorchidism, following vasectomy, drugs.	A low sperm count should be confirmed by sending two other appropriately collected semen specimens for evaluation. Ref: Fertil Steril 1975;26:492.
Sjögren's antibodies, serum (SS-A) Negative Marbled $$$	Sjögren's syndrome antibody (SS-A) is an antibody against acidic nuclear ribonucleoproteins that is found in patients with some connective tissue diseases, especially Sjögren's syndrome. (See also Autoantibodies table, p 226.)	**Positive in:** Primary Sjögren's syndrome (70%), SLE (40%), rheumatoid arthritis (10%).	Patients with antibodies to SS-A may have a negative ANA test. Anti-La/SS-B is another antibody against acidic ribonucleoproteins that is less sensitive for Sjögren's (50-60%) and SLE (10-15%). Ref: Arthritis Rheum 1980;23:287. Ref: Semin Arthritis Rheum 1987; 16:237.

	Smooth muscle Abs	Sodium
Smooth muscle antibodies, serum Negative Marbled $$	Detects antibodies against smooth muscle proteins, found in patients with chronic active hepatitis and primary biliary cirrhosis.	**Positive in:** Autoimmune chronic active hepatitis (40–70%, predominantly IgG antibodies), lower titers in primary biliary cirrhosis (50%, predominantly IgM antibodies), viral hepatitis, infectious mononucleosis, cryptogenic cirrhosis (28%), < 2% of normal individuals.	The presence of high titers of smooth muscle antibodies (> 1:80) is useful in distinguishing autoimmune chronic active hepatitis from other forms of hepatitis. Ref: Gut 1980;21:878.
Sodium, serum (Na$^+$) 135–145 meq/L [mmol/L] *Panic:* < 125 or > 155 meq/L Marbled $	Sodium is the predominant extracellular cation. The serum sodium level is primarily determined by the volume status of the individual. Hyponatremia can be divided into hypovolemia, euvolemia, and hypervolemia categories (see Hyponatremia algorithm, p 254).	**Increased in:** Dehydration (excessive sweating, severe vomiting or diarrhea), polyuria (diabetes mellitus, diabetes insipidus), hyperaldosteronism, inadequate water intake (coma, hypothalamic disease). Drugs: steroids, licorice, oral contraceptives. **Decreased in:** Congestive heart failure, cirrhosis, vomiting, diarrhea, excessive sweating (with replacement of water but not salt), salt-losing nephropathy, adrenal insufficiency, nephrotic syndrome, water intoxication, SIADH. Drugs: thiazides, diuretics, ACE inhibitors, chlorpropamide, carbamazepine.	Spurious hyponatremia may be produced by severe lipemia or hyperproteinemia if sodium analysis involves a dilution step. The serum sodium falls about 1.6 meq/L for each 100 mg/dL increase in blood glucose. Hyponatremia in a normovolemic patient with urine osmolality higher than plasma osmolality suggests the possibility of SIADH, myxedema, hypopituitarism, or reset osmostat. Ref: Am J Med 1982;72:496. Ref: Ann Intern Med 1985;102:164.

Somatomedin C			
Test/Range/Collection	Physiologic Basis	Interpretation (sensitivity)	Comments
Somatomedin C, plasma 123–463 ng/mL (age- and sex-dependent) Lavender $$$$	Somatomedin C is a growth hormone-dependent plasma peptide produced by the liver. It is believed to mediate the growth-promoting effect of growth hormone (GH). It has an anabolic, insulin-like action on fat and muscle and stimulates collagen and protein synthesis. Its level is relatively constant throughout the day.	**Increased in:** Acromegaly (level correlates with disease activity better than GH level). **Decreased in:** Pituitary dwarfism, hypopituitarism, Laron dwarfism (end-organ resistance to GH), fasting for 5–6 days, poor nutrition, hypothyroidism, cirrhosis. Values may be normal in growth hormone-deficient patients with hyperprolactinemia or craniopharyngioma.	A normal somatomedin C level in children is strong evidence that GH deficiency is not present and precludes the need for extensive pituitary function testing. A low level does not prove that GH deficiency is present, since levels may be reduced in malnutrition, malabsorption, chronic systemic illness, and hypothyroidism. Reference range here is for an immunoassay done following displacement of somatomedin C from its binding protein (acid-ethanol extraction). Ref: J Clin Endocrinol 1988;66:538. Ref: N Engl J Med 1979;301:1138. Ref: J Pediatr 1981;99:720.

	Testosterone	**Thrombin time**
Testosterone, serum Males: 3.0–10.0 ng/mL Females: 0.3–0.7 ng/mL [Males: 10–35 nmol/L Females: 1.0–2.4 nmol/L] Marbled $$$	Testosterone is the principal male sex hormone, produced by the Leydig cells of the testes. In serum, it is largely bound to albumin (38%) and to a specific steroid hormone-binding globulin (60%), but it is the free hormone (2%) that is physiologically active. Unless otherwise specified, the total testosterone level measures both bound and free testosterone in the serum (by immunoassay).	**Increased in:** Idiopathic sexual precocity (in boys, levels may be in adult range), adrenal hyperplasia (boys), adrenocortical tumors, trophoblastic disease during pregnancy, idiopathic hirsutism, arrhenoblastoma, virilizing ovarian tumors, virilizing luteoma, testicular feminization (normal or moderately elevated). Drugs: anticonvulsants, barbiturates, estrogens, oral contraceptives (through increased binding globulin). **Decreased in:** Hypogonadism (primary and secondary, orchidectomy, Klinefelter's, uremia, hepatic insufficiency, ethanol [men]). Drugs: digoxin, spironolactone.	Serum testosterone levels decrease in men after age 50. A free testosterone level is indicated when a normal total testosterone level is thought not to reflect free testosterone levels because of increases in steroid hormone-binding globulin. Ref: N Engl J Med 1980;303:682.
Thrombin time, plasma 24–35 seconds (laboratory-specific) Blue $	Prolongation of the thrombin time indicates a defect in conversion of fibrinogen to fibrin.	**Increased in:** Low fibrinogen (< 50 mg/dL), abnormal fibrinogen (dysfibrinogenemia), increased fibrin degradation products (eg, disseminated intravascular coagulation), heparin, fibrinolytic agents (streptokinase, urokinase, tissue plasminogen activator).	Thrombin time can be used to monitor fibrinolytic therapy and to screen for dysfibrinogenemia or circulating anticoagulants.

Test/Range/Collection	Physiologic Basis	Interpretation (sensitivity)	Comments
Thyroglobulin		
Thyroglobulin, serum 3–42 ng/mL [μg/L] Marbled $$$	Thyroglobulin is a large protein specific to the thyroid gland from which thyroxine is synthesized and cleaved.	**Increased in:** Hyperthyroidism, subacute thyroiditis, untreated thyroid carcinomas (except medullary carcinoma). **Decreased in:** Factitious hyperthyroidism, presence of thyroglobulin autoantibodies, after total thyroidectomy.	Thyroglobulin is useful to follow patients after treatment of nonmedullary thyroid carcinomas. Levels fall after successful therapy and rise when metastases develop. Sensitivity of the test is increased if patients are off thyroid replacement for 6 weeks prior to testing or if given T_3 (Cytomel) for the first 4 weeks, then no medication for the last 2 weeks. Athyrotic patients on T_4 (L-thyroxine) should have values < 5 ng/mL and those off T_4 should have values < 10 ng/mL. Ref: Cancer 1983;52:1856. Ref: JAMA 1983;250:2352.
Thyroglobulin antibodies		
Thyroglobulin antibody, serum < 1:10 (highly method-dependent) Marbled $$	Antibodies against thyroglobulin are produced in autoimmune diseases of the thyroid and other organs. 10% of the normal population have slightly elevated titers (especially women and the elderly).	**Increased in:** Hashimoto's thyroiditis (> 90%), thyroid carcinoma (45%), thyrotoxicosis, pernicious anemia (50%), SLE (20%), subacute thyroiditis, Graves' disease. **Not increased in:** Multinodular goiter, thyroid adenomas, and some carcinomas.	The thyroid microsomal antibody test is more sensitive than the thyroglobulin antibody test in autoimmune thyroid disease. Absence of both makes autoimmune thyroid disease unlikely. A normal titer of thyroglobulin antibody does not exclude Hashimoto's thyroiditis. There is little indication for this test. If evidence for autoimmune thyroid disease is required, the more sensitive antimicrosomal antibody test should be ordered (see Thyroid microsomal antibodies, below). Ref: Am J Med 1983;74:941. Ref: Med Clin North Am 1991;75:1.

	Test	Physiology / Description	Interpretation	Comments
Thyroid microsomal Abs	**Thyroid microsomal antibody**, serum Negative (highly method-dependent) Marbled $$	Test detects antibodies to microsomal antigens of thyroid epithelial cells produced in autoimmune disease of thyroid and other organs.	**Increased in:** Hashimoto's thyroiditis (> 90%), Graves' disease, few thyroid carcinomas, SLE, pernicious anemia, some normal women over 40 years old. **Not increased in:** Multinodular goiter, most thyroid adenomas or carcinomas.	Test is indicated to confirm clinical impression of autoimmune thyroid disease. It is not a measure of thyroid function. Test is more sensitive than thyroglobulin antibody test but is not specific for autoimmune thyroid disease. Ref: Am J Med 1983;74:941. Ref: Med Clin North Am 1991;75:1.
Thyroid-stimulating hormone	**Thyroid-stimulating hormone**, serum (TSH) 0.4–6 μU/mL [mU/L] Marbled $$	TSH is an anterior pituitary hormone that stimulates the thyroid gland to produce thyroid hormones. Secretion is stimulated by thyrotropin-releasing hormone from the hypothalamus. There is negative feedback on TSH secretion from circulating thyroid hormone.	**Increased in:** Hypothyroidism. Mild increases in recovery phase of acute illness. **Decreased in:** Hyperthyroidism, acute medical or surgical illness, pituitary hypothyroidism. Drugs: dopamine, high-dose corticosteroids.	Newly developed sensitive assays can detect low enough levels of TSH to be useful in the diagnosis of hyperthyroidism as well as hypothyroidism. (See also Thyroid function table, p 242.) Test is useful for following patients taking thyroid medication. Neonatal and cord blood levels are 2–4 times higher than adult levels. Ref: J Nucl Med 1985;26:1248.

Test/Range/Collection	Physiologic Basis	Interpretation (sensitivity)	Comments
Thyroid-stimulating immunoglobulin, serum (TSI) < 130% basal activity of adenylyl cyclase Marbled $$$$	Test detects heterogeneous IgG antibodies directed against the TSH receptor on thyroid cells. Frequently, they cause excess release of hormone from the thyroid. Test measures antibodies indirectly by how much they stimulate adenylyl cyclase to produce cAMP.	**Increased in:** Graves' disease.	Although TSI is a marker of Graves' disease, the test is not necessary for the diagnosis in most cases. Test is very rarely indicated but may be helpful in (1) pregnant women with a history of Graves' disease, because TSI may have some predictive value for neonatal thyrotoxicosis; (2) patients presenting with exophthalmos who are euthyroid, to confirm Graves' disease. Use of the test to predict relapse of hyperthyroidism at the end of a course of antithyroid drugs is controversial. Ref: J Clin Endocrinol Metab 1989; 69:1093.
Thyroxine, total, serum (T_4) 5.0–11.0 µg/dL [64–142 nmol/L] Marbled $	Total T_4 is a measure of thyroid gland secretion of T_4, bound and free, and thus is influenced by serum thyroid hormone binding activity.	**Increased in:** Hyperthyroidism, increased thyroid binding globulin (TBG) (eg, pregnancy, drug). Drugs: amiodarone, high-dose beta-blockers (especially propranolol). **Decreased in:** Hypothyroidism, low TBG due to illness or drugs, congenital absence of TBG. Drugs: phenytoin, carbamazepine, androgens.	Total T_4 should be interpreted with the TBG level or as part of a free thyroxine index. Ref: Med Clin North Am 1991;75:1. Ref: Med Clin North Am 1991;75:27.

Table header: Thyroid-stimulating immunoglobulin / Thyroxine (T_4), total

			Thyroxine, free	Thyroxine index, free
Thyroxine, free, serum (FT$_4$) Varies with method Marbled $$		FT$_4$ (if done by equilibrium dialysis or ultrafiltration method) is a more direct measure of the free T$_4$ hormone concentration (biologically available hormone) than the free T$_4$ index. FT$_4$ done by a 2-step immunoassay is similar to the free thyroxine index.	**Increased in:** Hyperthyroidism, nonthyroidal illness, especially psychiatric. Drugs: amiodarone, beta-blockers (high dose). **Decreased in:** Hypothyroidism, nonthyroidal illness. Drugs: phenytoin.	FT$_4$ index is functionally equivalent to the FT$_4$ (see Thyroxine index, free, below). (See also Thyroid function table, p 242.)
Thyroxine index, free, serum (FT$_4$I) 6.5–12.5 Marbled $$		Free thyroxine index is expressed as total T$_4$ × T$_3$ (or T$_4$) resin uptake and provides an estimate of the level of free T$_4$, since the T$_3$ (or T$_4$) resin uptake (ie, thyroid hormone binding ratio) is an indirect estimate of the thyroid binding globulin (TBG) concentration. (TBG binds 70% of circulating thyroid hormone.) The unbound form of circulating T$_4$, normally 0.03% of total serum T$_4$, determines the amount of T$_4$ available to cells.	**Increased in:** Hyperthyroidism, nonthyroidal illness, especially psychiatric. Drugs: amiodarone, beta-blockers (high dose). **Decreased in:** Hypothyroidism, nonthyroidal illness. Drugs: phenytoin.	FT$_4$I is functionally equivalent to the Thyroxine, free (see Thyroxine, free, above). Test is useful in patients with clinically suspected hyper- or hypothyroidism, in elderly patients admitted to geriatric units, or in women over 40 with one or more somatic complaints. (See Thyroid function table, p 242.) Screening for thyroid disease is not indicated in younger women, men, or patients admitted with acute medical or psychiatric illnesses because transient abnormalities are indistinguishable from true thyroid disease. Ref: Ann Intern Med 1990;112:840.

	***Toxoplasma* antibody**		
Test/Range/Collection	**Physiologic Basis**	**Interpretation (sensitivity)**	**Comments**
***Toxoplasma* anti-body**, serum or CSF (Toxo) IgG: < 1:16 IgM: Infant < 1:2 Adult < 1:8 titer Marbled or CSF $$$ Submit paired sera, one collected within 1 week of illness and another 2–3 weeks later.	*Toxoplasma gondii* is an obligate intracellular protozoan that causes human infection via ingestion, transplacental transfer, blood products, or organ transplantation. In the immunodeficient host, acute infection may progress to lethal encephalitis, pneumonitis, or myocarditis. In acute primary infection, IgM antibodies develop 1–2 weeks after onset of illness, peak in 6–8 weeks, and then decline. IgG antibodies develop on a similar timecourse but persist for years. In adult infection, the disease usually represents a reactivation, not a primary infection. Therefore, the IgM test is less useful.	**Increased in:** Acute or congenital toxoplasmosis (IgM), previous *Toxoplasma* exposure (IgG), and false-positive reactions (SLE, rheumatoid arthritis).	Approximately 30% of all US adults have antibodies to *T gondii*. Single IgG titers of > 1:256 are considered diagnostic of active infection; titers of > 1:128 are suspicious. Titers of 1:16–1:64 may merely represent past exposure, but if titers subsequently rise, they probably represent early disease. IgM titer >1:16 is very important in the diagnosis of congenital toxoplasmosis. High titer IgG antibody results should prompt an IgM test. IgM, however, is generally not found in adult AIDS patients since the disease usually represents a reactivation. Some recommend ordering baseline *Toxoplasma* IgG titers in all asymptomatic HIV-positive patients because if neurologic signs and symptoms develop in the future, a rising *Toxoplasma* titer can help diagnose CNS toxoplasmosis. (See also Brain abscess, p 151.) Ref: N Engl J Med 1988;318:271. Ref: Ann Intern Med 1984;100:36.

	Triglycerides	Triiodothyronine (T$_3$)
Triglycerides, serum (Tg) < 165 mg/dL [< 1.65 g/L] Marbled $ Fasting specimen required.	Dietary fat is hydrolyzed in the small intestine, absorbed and resynthesized by mucosal cells, and secreted into lacteals as chylomicrons. Triglycerides in the chylomicrons are cleared from the blood by tissue lipoprotein lipase. Endogenous triglyceride production occurs in the liver. These triglycerides are transported in association with β-lipoproteins in very low density lipoproteins (VLDL).	**Increased in:** Hypothyroidism, diabetes mellitus, nephrotic syndrome, chronic alcoholism (fatty liver), biliary tract obstruction, stress, familial lipoprotein lipase deficiency, familial dysbetalipoproteinemia, familial combined hyperlipidemia, obesity, viral hepatitis, cirrhosis, pancreatitis, chronic renal failure, gout, pregnancy, glycogen storage diseases types I, III, and VI, anorexia nervosa, dietary excess. Drugs: beta-blockers, cholestyramine, corticosteroids, diazepam, diuretics, estrogens, oral contraceptives. **Decreased in:** Tangier disease (α-lipoprotein deficiency), hypo- and abetalipoproteinemia, malnutrition, malabsorption, parenchymal liver disease, hyperthyroidism, intestinal lymphangiectasia. Drugs: ascorbic acid, clofibrate, nicotinic acid, gemfibrozil.	If serum is clear, the serum triglyceride level is generally < 350 mg/dL. Hypertriglyceridemia in an asymptomatic person who does not have a strong family history of coronary heart disease or a personal history of hypercholesterolemia is not a definite risk factor for coronary heart disease. Ref: Ann Intern Med 1989;110:622.
Triiodothyronine, total, serum (T$_3$) 95–190 ng/dL [1.5–2.9 nmol/L] Marbled $$	T$_3$ reflects the metabolically active form of thyroid hormone and is influenced by thyroid hormone binding activity.	**Increased in:** Hyperthyroidism (some), increased thyroid binding globulin. **Decreased in:** Hypothyroidism, nonthyroidal illness, decreased thyroid binding globulin.	Test may be increased in approximately 5% of hyperthyroid patients in whom T$_4$ is normal (T$_3$ toxicosis). Therefore, test is indicated when hyperthyroidism is suspected and T$_4$ value is normal. Test is of no value in the diagnosis of hypothyroidism. Ref: Ann Intern Med 1990;112:840.

Test/Range/Collection	Physiologic Basis	Interpretation (sensitivity)	Comments
		Tularemia agglutinins	
Tularemia agglutinins, serum < 1:80 titer Marbled $$	*Francisella tularensis* is an organism of wild rodents that infects humans (eg, trappers and skinners) via contact with animal tissues, by the bite of certain ticks and flies, and by consumption of undercooked meat or contaminated water. Agglutinins appear in 10–14 days and peak in 5–10 weeks. Titers decrease over years.	**Increased in:** Tularemia; cross-reaction with *Brucella* antigens and *Proteus* OX-19 antigen (but at lower titers).	Titers of > 1:160 are indicative of infection. Maximum titers are > 1:1280. A history of exposure to rabbits, ticks, dogs, cats, or skunks is suggestive of, but is not a requirement for, the diagnosis. Culture of the organism is difficult and hazardous to laboratory personnel. Serologic tests are the mainstay of diagnosis. Ref: Medicine 1985;64:251.
		Type and screen	
Type and screen, serum and red cells Red or lavender $$ Specimen label must be signed by the person drawing the blood. A second "check" specimen is needed at some hospitals.	Type and screen includes ABO and Rh grouping (see pp 41 and 123, respectively) and antibody screen (see p 48). (Compare with Type and cross-match, below.)		Type and screen is indicated for patients undergoing operative procedures unlikely to require transfusion. A negative antibody screen implies that a recipient can receive un-cross-matched type-specific blood with minimal risk. If the recipient's serum contains a clinically significant alloantibody by antibody screen, a cross-match is required. Ref: *Technical Manual of the American Association of Blood Banks*, 10th ed. American Association of Blood Banks, 1990.

	Type and cross-match	Uric acid
Type and cross-match, serum and red cells (Type and cross) Red or lavender $$ Specimen label must be signed by the person drawing the blood. A second "check" specimen is needed at some hospitals.	A type and cross-match involves ABO and Rh grouping (see pp 41 and 123, respectively), antibody screen (see p 48), and cross-match. (Compare with Type and screen, above.) A major cross-match involves testing recipient serum against donor cells. It uses antihuman globulin to detect recipient's antibodies on donor red cells. If the recipient's serum contains a clinically significant alloantibody by antibody screen, a cross-match is required.	A type and screen is adequate preparation for operative procedures unlikely to require transfusion. Unnecessary type and cross-match orders reduce blood availability and add to costs. In addition, a preordering system should be in place, indicating the number of units of blood likely to be needed for each operative procedure. Ref: *Technical Manual of the American Association of Blood Banks*, 10th ed. American Association of Blood Banks, 1990.
Uric acid, serum Males: 2.4–7.4 Females 1.4–5.8 mg/dL [Males: 140–440 Females: 80–350 μmol/L] Marbled $	Uric acid is an end product of nucleoprotein metabolism and is excreted by the kidney. An increase in serum uric acid concentration occurs with increased nucleoprotein synthesis or catabolism (blood dyscrasias, therapy of leukemia) or decreased renal uric acid excretion (eg, thiazide diuretic therapy or renal failure).	**Increased in:** Renal failure, gout, myeloproliferative disorders (leukemia, lymphoma, myeloma, polycythemia vera), psoriasis, glycogen storage disease (type I), Lesch-Nyhan syndrome (X-linked hypoxanthine-guanine phosphoribosyltransferase deficiency), lead nephropathy. Drugs: antimetabolite and chemotherapeutic agents, diuretics, ethanol, nicotinic acid, salicylates (low dose). **Decreased in:** SIADH, xanthine oxidase deficiency, low-purine diet, Fanconi's syndrome, neoplastic disease (various, causing increased renal excretion), liver disease. Drugs: salicylates (high dose), allopurinol (xanthine oxidase inhibitor). Sex and age affect uric acid levels. The incidence of hyperuricemia is greater in some racial groups (eg, Filipinos) than others (whites). Ref: Am J Med 1987;82:421. Ref: Ann Intern Med 1973;78:239.

Test/Range/Collection	Physiologic Basis	Interpretation (sensitivity)	Comments
	Vanillylmandelic acid		**VDRL, serum**
Vanillylmandelic acid, urine (VMA) 2–7 mg/24 h [10–35 μmol/d] Urine bottle containing hydrochloric acid $$ Collect 24-hour urine.	Catecholamines secreted in excess by pheochromocytomas are metabolized by the enzymes monoamine oxidase and catechol-O-methyltransferase to VMA, which is excreted in urine.	**Increased in:** Pheochromocytoma (96%, 100% specificity), neuroblastoma, ganglioneuroma. **Decreased in:** Drugs: monoamine oxidase inhibitors.	A 24-hour urine metanephrine test (p 106) is the recommended test for the diagnosis of pheochromocytoma. (See also Pheochromocytoma algorithm, p 256.) A special diet is not needed when VMA test is done by the usual method. < 0.1% of hypertensive patients have a pheochromocytoma. Ref: Am J Cardiol 1970;26:270. Ref: Ann Surg 1974;179:740.
Venereal Disease Research Laboratory test, serum (VDRL) Nonreactive Marbled $	Measures nontreponemal antibodies that are produced when *Treponema pallidum* interacts with host tissues. The VDRL usually turns reactive at a titer of > 1:32 within 1–3 weeks after the genital chancre appears.	**Increased in:** Syphilis: primary (59–87%), secondary (100%), late latent (79–91%), tertiary (37–94%); collagen-vascular diseases (rheumatoid arthritis, SLE), infections (mononucleosis, leprosy, malaria), pregnancy, drug abuse.	VDRL is used as a screening test and in suspected cases of primary and secondary syphilis. Positive tests should be confirmed with an FTA-ABS or MHA-TP test (see pp 80 and 108, respectively). The VDRL has similar sensitivity and specificity to the RPR (see Syphilis test table, p 240). Ref: Ann Intern Med 1991;114:1005. Ref: Ann Intern Med 1986;104:368.

	VDRL, CSF	Vitamin B$_{12}$
Venereal Disease Research Laboratory test, CSF (VDRL) Nonreactive $$ Deliver in a clean plastic or glass tube.	The CSF VDRL measures nontreponemal antibodies that develop in the CSF when *Treponema pallidum* interacts with the central nervous system.	The quantitative VDRL is the test of choice for CNS syphilis. Treponemal tests (FTA-ABS, MHA-TP) are not helpful in CSF. Since the sensitivity of CSF VDRL is very low, a negative test does not rule out neurosyphilis. Clinical features, CSF white cell count, and CSF protein should be used together to make the diagnosis (see CSF profiles, p 228). Because the specificity of the CSF VDRL test is high, a positive test confirms the presence of neurosyphilis. Ref: Neurology 1985;35:1368. Ref: West J Med 1988;149:47.
	Increased in: Tertiary neurosyphilis (10%).	
Vitamin B$_{12}$, serum 140–820 pg/mL [100–600 pmol/L] Marbled $$	Vitamin B$_{12}$ is a necessary cofactor for 2 important biochemical processes: conversion of methylmalonyl-CoA to succinyl-CoA and methylation of homocysteine to methionine. All vitamin B$_{12}$ comes from ingestion of foods of animal origin. Vitamin B$_{12}$ in serum is protein-bound, 70% to transcobalamin I (TC I) and 30% to transcobalamin II (TC II). The B$_{12}$ bound to TC II is physiologically active; that bound to TC I is not.	Confirmation of suspected vitamin B$_{12}$ deficiency requires a vitamin B$_{12}$ absorption (Schilling's) test (see below). The commonly available competitive protein binding assay measures total B$_{12}$. It is insensitive to significant decreases in physiologically significant B$_{12}$ bound to TC II. Specificity of the serum vitamin B$_{12}$ test (approximately 73%) has not been systematically studied. Neuropsychiatric disorders caused by low serum B$_{12}$ level can occur in the absence of anemia or macrocytosis. Ref: Am J Med 1987;82:291. Ref: Geriatrics 1988;43(3):89.
	Increased in: Leukemia (acute myelocytic, chronic myelocytic, chronic lymphocytic, monocytic), marked leukocytosis, polycythemia vera. (Increased B$_{12}$ levels are not diagnostically useful.) **Decreased in:** Pernicious anemia, gastrectomy, gastric carcinoma, malabsorption (sprue, celiac disease, steatorrhea, regional enteritis, fistulas, bowel resection, *Diphyllobothrium latum* [fish tapeworm] infestation, small bowel bacterial overgrowth), pregnancy, dietary deficiency, drugs.	

Test/Range/Collection	Physiologic Basis	Interpretation (sensitivity)	Comments
Vitamin B_{12} absorption test			
Vitamin B_{12} absorption test, 24-hour urine (Schilling's test) Excretion of > 8% of administered dose $$$$ Stage I: 0.5–1.0 μCi of ^{57}Co-B_{12} is given orally and then 1.0 mg of unlabeled B_{12} is given IM 2 hours later. A 24-hour urine is collected. Stage II: After 5 days, test is repeated with 60 mg active hog intrinsic factor added to the oral radioactive-labeled B_{12}.	Absorption of vitamin B_{12} is dependent on 2 factors: adequate intrinsic factor produced by the stomach antrum and normal ileal absorption. Lack of either can lead to B_{12} deficiency.	**Decreased in:** Ileal disease or resection, bacterial overgrowth, B_{12} deficiency (because megaloblastosis of the intestinal wall leads to decreased B_{12} absorption), pernicious anemia (<2.5% excretion of administered dose), postgastrectomy, chronic pancreatitis, cystic fibrosis, giardiasis, Crohn's disease.	If the patient's creatinine clearance is < 60 mL/min, a 48-hour urine should be collected. Pernicious anemia is suggested by an abnormal stage I test, followed by a normal stage II test (ie, addition of intrinsic factor leads to normal intestinal absorption and urinary excretion). Ileal malabsorption gives abnormal results in stages I and II. Ref: CRC Crit Rev Clin Lab Sci 1988; 26:263.

	Vitamin D, 25-hydroxy		
Vitamin D, 25-hydroxy, serum or plasma (25[OH]D) 10–50 ng/mL [25–125 nmol/L] Marbled or green $$$	The vitamin D system functions to maintain serum calcium levels. Vitamin D is a fat-soluble steroid hormone with two molecular forms: D_3 (cholecalciferol) and D_2 (ergocalciferol). To achieve biologic potency, both need to be further metabolized. Two sequential hydroxylations occur: in the liver to 25(OH)D and then, in the kidney, to 1,25-dihydroxy vitamin D. Plasma levels increase with sun exposure.	**Increased in:** Heavy milk drinkers (up to 64 ng/mL), vitamin D intoxication, sun exposure. **Decreased in:** Dietary deficiency, malabsorption (rickets, osteomalacia), biliary and portal cirrhosis, nephrotic syndrome, lack of sun exposure. Drugs: phenytoin, phenobarbital.	Measurement of 25(OH)D is the best indicator of both vitamin D deficiency and toxicity and is indicated in hypocalcemic disorders associated with increased PTH levels or in hypercalcemic disorders associated with decreased PTH levels. Ref: Adv Intern Med 1982;27:45.

	Vitamin D, 1,25-dihydroxy		
Vitamin D, 1,25-dihydroxy, serum or plasma (1,25[OH]$_2$D) 20–76 pg/mL Marbled or green $$$$	1,25-dihydroxy vitamin D is the most potent form of vitamin D. The main actions of vitamin D are the acceleration of calcium and phosphate absorption in the intestine and stimulation of bone resorption.	**Increased in:** Primary hyperparathyroidism, idiopathic hypercalciuria, sarcoidosis, some lymphomas, 1,25(OH)$_2$D-resistant rickets, normal growth (children), pregnancy, and lactation. **Decreased in:** Chronic renal failure, anephric patients, hypoparathyroidism, pseudohypoparathyroidism, 1α-hydroxylase deficiency, postmenopausal osteoporosis.	Test is rarely needed. Measurement of 1,25(OH)$_2$D is only useful in distinguishing 1α-hydroxylase deficiency from 1,25(OH)$_2$D-resistant rickets or in monitoring vitamin D status of patients with chronic renal failure. Test is not useful for assessment of vitamin D intoxication, because of efficient feedback regulation of 1,25(OH)$_2$D synthesis. Ref: Adv Intern Med 1982;27:45. Ref: N Engl J Med 1989;320:980.

Test/Range/Collection	Physiologic Basis	Interpretation (sensitivity)	Comments
von Willebrand factor			**von Willebrand factor**
von Willebrand's factor protein (immunologic), plasma (vWF) 44–158% Units Blue $$$	von Willebrand's factor (vWF) is produced by endothelial cells, circulates in the plasma complexed to factor VIII coagulant protein, and mediates platelet adhesion. Both quantitative and qualitative changes in vWF can cause disease. vWF can be measured as protein antigen (immunologic measure) or by ristocetin cofactor activity (functional assay).	**Increased in:** Inflammatory states (acute phase reactant). **Decreased in:** von Willebrand's disease.	In von Willebrand's disease, the platelet number and morphology are generally normal and the bleeding time is usually prolonged (markedly prolonged by aspirin). Variant forms associated with mild thrombocytopenia and angiodysplasia are described. The PTT may not be prolonged if factor VIII coagulant level is > 30%. Diagnosis is suggested by bleeding symptoms and family history. Ref: Blood 1987;70:895.
D-Xylose absorption test, urine > 5.0 g/5-hour urine (> 20% excreted in 5 hours) $$$ Fasting patient is given D-xylose, 25 g in 2 glasses of water, followed by 4 glasses of water over the next 2 hours. Urine is collected for 5 hours and refrigerated.	Xylose normally should be easily absorbed from the small intestine. Measuring xylose in serum or its excretion in urine after ingestion evaluates the carbohydrate absorption ability of the proximal small intestine.	**Decreased in:** Intestinal malabsorption, small intestinal bacterial overgrowth, renal insufficiency.	**D-Xylose absorption test** Test can be helpful in distinguishing intestinal malabsorption (decreased D-xylose absorption) from pancreatic insufficiency (normal D-xylose absorption). Urinary xylose excretion may be spuriously decreased in renal failure, thus limiting the specificity and usefulness of the test. In this case, a serum xylose level (gray top tube) obtained 1-hour after administration of a 25-g dose of D-xylose can be used to evaluate xylose absorption. The normal level should be > 29 mg/dL (1.9 mmol/L). Ref: Dig Dis Sci 1991;36:188.

4 Therapeutic Drug Monitoring: Principles & Test Interpretation

UNDERLYING ASSUMPTIONS

The basic assumptions underlying therapeutic drug monitoring are that drug metabolism varies from patient to patient and that the plasma level of a drug is more closely related to the drug's therapeutic effect or toxicity than is the dosage.

INDICATIONS FOR DRUG MONITORING

Drugs with a **narrow therapeutic index** (where therapeutic drug levels do not differ greatly from levels associated with serious toxicity) should be monitored. *Example*: Lithium.

Patients who have **impaired clearance** of a drug with a narrow therapeutic index are candidates for drug monitoring. The clearance mechanism of the drug involved must be known. *Example*: Patients with renal failure have decreased clearance of gentamicin and therefore are at a higher risk for gentamicin toxicity.

Drugs whose **toxicity is difficult to distinguish from a patient's underlying disease** may require monitoring. *Example*: Theophylline in patients with chronic obstructive pulmonary disease.

Drugs whose **efficacy is difficult to establish clinically** may require monitoring of plasma levels. *Example*: Phenytoin.

SITUATIONS IN WHICH DRUG MONITORING MAY NOT BE USEFUL

Drugs that can be given in extremely high doses before toxicity is apparent are not candidates for monitoring. *Example*: Penicillin.

If there are better means of assessing drug effects, drug level monitoring may not be appropriate. *Example*: Warfarin is monitored by prothrombin time determinations, not by serum levels.

Drug level monitoring to assess compliance is unreliable, since poor compliance cannot be distinguished from rapid metabolism without direct inpatient scrutiny of drug administration.

Drug toxicity cannot be diagnosed with drug levels alone; it is a clinical diagnosis. Drug levels within the usual therapeutic range do not rule out drug toxicity in a given patient. *Example*: Digoxin, where other physiologic variables (eg, hypokalemia) affect drug toxicity.

In summary, therapeutic drug monitoring may be useful to guide dosage adjustment of certain drugs in certain patients. Patient compliance is essential if drug monitoring data are to be correctly interpreted.

OTHER INFORMATION REQUIRED FOR EFFECTIVE DRUG MONITORING

Reliability of the Analytic Method

The **analytic sensitivity** of the drug monitoring method must be adequate. For some drugs, plasma levels are only in the ng/mL range. *Example*: Tricyclic antidepressants.

The **specificity** of the method must be known, since the drug's metabolites or other drugs may interfere. Interference by metabolites—which may or may not be pharmacologically active—is of particular concern in immunologic assay methods using antibodies to the parent drug.

The **precision** of the method must be known in order to assess whether changes in levels are caused by method imprecision or by clinical changes.

Reliability of the Therapeutic Range

Establishing the therapeutic range for a drug requires a reliable clinical assessment of its therapeutic and toxic effects, together with plasma drug level measurements by a particular analytic method. In practice, as newer, more specific analytic methods are introduced, the therapeutic ranges for those methods are estimated by comparing the old and new methodologies—without clinical correlation.

Pharmacokinetic Parameters

Five pharmacokinetic parameters that are important in therapeutic drug monitoring include:

1. *Bioavailability*. The bioavailability of a drug depends in part on its formulation. A drug that is significantly metabolized as it first passes through the liver exhibits a marked "first-pass effect," reducing the effective oral absorption of the drug. A reduction in this first-pass effect (eg, because of decreased hepatic blood flow in heart failure) could cause a clinically significant increase in effective oral drug absorption.

2. *Volume of distribution and distribution phases*. The volume of distribution of a drug determines the plasma concentration reached after a loading dose. The distribution phase is the time taken for a drug to distribute from the plasma to the periphery. Drug levels drawn before completion of a long distribution phase may not reflect levels of pharmacologically active drug at sites of action. *Examples*: Digoxin, lithium.

3. *Clearance*. Clearance is either renal or nonrenal (usually hepatic). Whereas changes in renal clearance can be predicted on the basis of serum creatinine or creatinine clearance, there is no routine liver function test for assessment of hepatic drug metabolism. For most therapeutic drugs measured, clearance is independent of plasma drug concentration, so that a change in dose is reflected in a similar change in plasma level. If, however, clearance is dose-dependent, dosage adjustments produce disproportionately large changes in plasma levels and must be made cautiously. *Example*: Phenytoin.

4. *Half-life*. The half-life of a drug depends on its volume of distribution and its clearance and determines the time taken to reach a steady state level. In 3 or 4 half-lives, the drug level will be 87.5% to 93.75% of the way to steady state. Patients with decreased drug clearance and therefore increased drug half-life will take longer to reach a higher steady state level. In general, since non-steady state drug levels are difficult to interpret, therapeutic drug monitoring usually involves measurement of drug levels at steady state.

5. *Protein binding of drugs*. All routine drug level analysis involves assessment of both protein-bound and free drug. However, pharmacologic activity depends on only the free drug level. Changes in protein binding (eg, in uremia or hypoalbuminemia) may significantly affect interpretation of reported levels for drugs that are highly protein-bound. *Example*: Phenytoin. In such cases, where the ratio of active to total measured drug level is increased, the therapeutic range based on total drug level will not apply.

Drug Interactions

For patients receiving several medications, the possibility of drug interactions affecting drug metabolism must be considered. *Example*: Quinidine decreases digoxin clearance.

Time to Draw Levels

In general, the specimen should be drawn after steady state is reached (at least 3 or 4 half-lives after a dosage adjustment) and just before the next dose (trough level).

Peak and trough levels may be indicated to evaluate the dosage of drugs whose half-lives are much shorter than the dosing interval. *Example*: Gentamicin.

Reference

Winter M: *Basic clinical pharmacokinetics*, 2nd ed. Applied Therapeutics, 1988.

Table 4-1. Therapeutic drug monitoring.

Drug	Effective Concentrations	Half-life (hours)	Dosage Adjustment	Comments
Amikacin	Peak: 10–25 µg/mL Trough: < 10 µg/mL	1–2.5, ↑ in uremia	↓ in renal dysfunction	Concomitant kanamycin or tobramycin therapy may give falsely elevated amikacin results by immunoassay.
Amitriptyline	160–240 ng/mL	9–161		Drug is highly protein-bound. Patient-specific decrease in protein binding may invalidate quoted range of effective concentration.
Carbamazepine	4–8 µg/mL	10–30		Induces its own metabolism. Metabolite 10,11-epoxide exhibits 13% cross-reactivity by immunoassay. Toxicity: diplopia, drowsiness, nausea, vomiting, and ataxia.
Desipramine	> 225 ng/mL	13–23		Drug is highly protein-bound. Patient-specific decrease in protein binding may invalidate quoted range of effective concentration.
Digoxin	0.8–2.0 ng/mL	42, ↑ in uremia, CHF, hypothyroidism; ↓ in hyperthyroidism	↓ in renal dysfunction, CHF	Bioavailability of digoxin tablets is 50–90%. Specimen must not be drawn within 6 hours of dose. Dialysis does not remove a significant amount. Hypokalemia potentiates toxicity. Digitalis toxicity is a clinical and *not* a laboratory diagnosis. Digibind (digoxin-specific antibody) therapy of digoxin overdose interferes with measurement of digoxin levels. Elimination reduced by quinidine and verapamil.
Gentamicin	Peak: 4–8 µg/mL Trough: < 2 µg/mL	2–5, ↑ in uremia (7.3 on dialysis)	↓ in renal dysfunction	Draw peak specimen 30 minutes after end of infusion. Draw trough just before next dose. In uremic patients, carbenicillin may ↓ gentamicin half-life from 46 to 22 hours.

Table 4–1 (cont'd). Therapeutic drug monitoring.

Drug	Effective Concentrations	Half-life (hours)	Dosage Adjustment	Comments
Imipramine	> 225 ng/mL	10–16		Drug is highly protein-bound. Patient-specific decrease in protein binding may invalidate quoted range of effective concentration.
Lidocaine	1–5 µg/mL	1.8, ↔ in uremia, CHF; ↑ in cirrhosis	↓ in CHF, liver disease	Levels increased with cimetidine therapy. CNS toxicity common in the elderly.
Lithium	0.7–2 meq/L	22, ↑ in uremia	↓ in renal dysfunction	Thiazides and loop diuretics may increase serum lithium levels.
Methotrexate		8.4, ↑ in uremia	↓ in renal dysfunction	7-OH methotrexate cross-reacts 1.5% in immunoassay. To minimize toxicity, leucovorin should be continued if methotrexate level is > 0.1 µmol/L at 48 hours after start of therapy. Methotrexate > 1 µmol/L at > 48 hrs requires an increase in leucovorin rescue therapy.
Nortriptyline	50–140 ng/mL	18–44		Drug is highly protein-bound. Patient-specific decrease in protein binding may invalidate quoted range of effective concentration.
Phenobarbital	10–30 µg/mL	86, ↑ in cirrhosis	↓ in liver disease	Metabolized primarily by the hepatic microsomal enzyme system. Many drug-drug interactions.

Table 4–1 (cont'd). Therapeutic drug monitoring.

Drug	Effective Concentrations	Half-life (hours)	Dosage Adjustment	Comments
Phenytoin	10–20 µg/mL ↓ in uremia, hypoalbuminemia	Dose-dependent		Metabolite cross-reacts 10% in immunoassay. Metabolism is capacity limited. Increase dose *cautiously* when level approaches therapeutic range, since new steady state level may be disproportionately higher. Drug is very highly protein-bound and when protein binding is decreased in uremia and hypoalbuminemia, usual therapeutic range does not apply. In this situation, use a reference range of 5–10 µg/mL.
Primidone	5–10 µg/mL	8		Phenobarbital cross-reacts 0.5%. Metabolized to phenobarbital. Primidone/phenobarbital ratio > 1:2 suggests poor compliance.
Procainamide	4–8 µg/mL	3, ↑ in uremia	↓ in renal dysfunction	30% of patients with plasma levels of 12–16 µg/mL have ECG changes; 40% of patients with plasma levels of 16 µg/mL have severe toxicity. Metabolite N-acetylprocainamide is active.
Quinidine	1–4 µg/mL	7, ↔ in CHF; ↑ in liver disease	↓ in liver disease, CHF	Effective concentration is lower in chronic liver disease and nephrosis where binding is decreased.
Salicylate	150–300 µg/mL (15–30 mg/dL)	Dose-dependent		See p 272 for nomogram of salicylate toxicity.
Theophylline	10–20 µg/mL	9	↓ in CHF, cirrhosis, and with cimetidine	Caffeine cross-reacts 10%. Elimination is increased 1.5–2.0 times in smokers. 1,3-dimethyl uric acid metabolite ↑ in uremia and because of cross-reactivity may cause an apparent slight ↑ in serum theophylline.
Tobramycin	Peak: 5–10 µg/mL Trough: < 2 µg/mL	2, ↑ in uremia	↓ in renal dysfunction	Tobramycin, kanamycin, and amikacin may cross-react in immunoassay.

5 Microbiology: Test Selection & Treatment

HOW TO USE THIS SECTION

This section displays information about clinically important infectious diseases in tabular form. Included in these tables are the *Organisms* involved in the disease/syndrome listed; *Specimens/Diagnostic Tests* that are useful in the evaluation; *Therapy* recommendations; and *Comments* regarding the tests and diagnoses discussed. Topics are listed by body area/organ system: Central Nervous System, Eye, Ear, Sinus, Upper Airway, Lung, Heart and Vessels, Abdomen, Genitourinary, Bone, Joint, Muscle, Skin, and Blood.

Organisms

This column lists organisms that are known to cause the stated illness. Scientific names are abbreviated according to common usage (eg, *Streptococcus pneumoniae* as *S pneumoniae* or pneumococcus). Specific age or risk groups are listed in order of increasing age and frequency (eg, Infant, Child, Adult, AIDS).

When bacteria are listed, Gram's stain characteristics follow the organism name in parentheses—eg, "*S pneumoniae* (GPDC)." The following abbreviations are used:

GPC	Gram-positive cocci	**GNC**	Gram-negative cocci
GPDC	Gram-positive diplococci	**GNDC**	Gram-negative diplococci
GPCB	Gram-positive coccobacilli	**GNCB**	Gram-negative coccobacilli
GPR	Gram-positive rods	**GNR**	Gram-negative rods
GVCB	Gram-variable coccobacilli	**AFB**	Acid-fast bacilli

When known, the frequency of the specific organism's involvement in the disease process is also provided in parentheses — eg, "*S pneumoniae* (GPDC) (50%)."

Specimen Collection/Diagnostic Tests

This column describes the collection of specimens, laboratory processing, useful radiographic procedures, and other diagnostic tests. Culture or test sensitivities with respect to the diagnosis in question are placed in parentheses immediately following the test when known — eg, "Gram's stain (60%)." Pertinent serologic tests are also listed. Keep in mind that few infections can be identified by definitive diagnostic tests and that clinical judgement is critical to making difficult diagnoses when test results are equivocal.

Therapy

Therapeutic recommendations use the following abbreviations:

Abbreviation	Drug	Abbreviation	Drug
Pen	Penicillin	Ceph 1	1st generation cephalosporin
HD	> 12–24 million units/d	Ceph 2	2nd generation cephalosporin
MD	8–12 million units/d	Ceph 3	3rd generation cephalosporin
AMP/X	Ampicillin or Amoxicillin	TMP/SMX	Trimethoprim/ sulfamethoxazole
APPen	Antipseudomonal penicillin		
PRPen	Penicillinase-resistant penicillin	AG	Aminoglycosides
		APAG	Antipseudomonal aminoglycoside
TC/CL	Ticarcillin/clavulanate		
AM/SB	Ampicillin/sulbactam		
AM/CL	Amoxicillin/clavulanate		
Vanc	Vancomycin	Aztr	Aztreonam
IMP/CIL	Imipenem/cilastin	FQ	Fluoroquinolones
Metr	Metronidazole	Cipr	Ciprofloxacin
Clinda	Clindamycin		
Tcn	Tetracycline	Ampho	Amphotericin B
Eryth	Erythromycin	Fluco	Fluconazole
		5FC	Flucytosine
PO	Oral		
IV	Intravenous	INH	Isoniazid
IM	Intramuscular	Rif	Rifampin
q	Every	PZA	Pyrazinamide
h	Hour	EMB	Ethambutol

Antibiotic combinations are shown with "+" signs, and alternative regimens are separated by "/" or "or." The therapeutic options recommended are empiric ones and should be used only as initial therapy while awaiting identification of specific causative organisms and their antibiotic sensitivities. Many of these therapeutic recommendations have been adapted and reproduced, with permission, from Sanford JP:

Guide to Antimicrobial Therapy 1991
Antimicrobial Therapy, Inc
5910 N Central Expressway
Dallas, Texas 75206

Comments

This column includes general information about the utility of the tests and may include useful information about patient management. Appropriate general references are also listed.

Syndrome Name/Body Area

In the last 2 columns the syndrome name and body area are placed perpendicular to the rest of the table to allow for quick referencing.

	CENTRAL NERVOUS SYSTEM		
	Brain Abscess		
Organism	**Specimens/Diagnostic Tests**	**Therapy**	**Comments**
Brain Abscess Usually polymicrobial: Viridans group and anaerobic streptococci (GPC in chains) (60–70%), *Bacteroides* (20–40%), Enterobacteriaceae (GNR) (23–33%), *S aureus* (GPC) (10–15%), fungus (10–15%), cysticercosis. HIV infection: *Toxoplasma gondii.* Post-traumatic: *S aureus* (GPC), Enterobacteriaceae (GNR).	Blood for bacterial cultures (aerobic and anaerobic). Brain abscess aspirate for bacterial, AFB, fungal cultures, and cytology. Lumbar puncture is nonspecific. CSF profile is potentially dangerous. Sources of infection in the ears, sinuses, lungs or bloodstream should be sought for culture when abscess is found. CT scan is the most valuable imaging procedure and can guide biopsy if a specimen is needed. (See CT scan of head, p. 192.) Serum *Toxoplasma* antibody in HIV-infected patients may not be positive at outset of presumptive therapy. If negative or if no response to empiric therapy, biopsy may be needed to rule out lymphoma or tuberculosis. (See also *Toxoplasma* antibody, p 134.)	Adult: PRPen + Ceph 3 + Metr or Pen + Metr or Pen + chloramphenicol.* *Toxoplasma* infection: Sulfadiazine + pyrimethamine.* Post-traumatic: PRPen + Ceph 3 + Rif or Vanc + Ceph 3 + Rif.* If CT scan shows cerebritis and patient is neurologically stable, antibiotics alone may be sufficient. However, deterioration in neurologic status mandates surgical drainage. Usually, bacteriologic diagnosis is presumptive, and therapy can begin once lesion is visualized.	Common in patients with cyanotic congenital heart disease and right-to-left shunting (eg, tetralogy of Fallot) or arteriovenous vascular abnormalities of the lung (eg, Osler-Weber-Rendu). Majority of toxoplasmosis abscesses are multiple and are best seen on MRI in the basal ganglia, parietal and frontal lobes. ^{99m}Technetium brain scan is a very sensitive test for abscess and the test of choice where CT or MRI are unavailable. Ref: J Neurosurg 1983;59: 972.

*Adapted and reproduced, with permission, from Sanford JP: *Guide to Antimicrobial Therapy 1991,* Antimicrobial Therapy, Inc, 1991.

	CENTRAL NERVOUS SYSTEM		
	Encephalitis		
Organism	**Specimens/Diagnostic Tests**	**Therapy**	**Comments**
Encephalitis Arboviruses (California, St. Louis, western equine), enteroviruses (coxsackie, echo, polio), herpes simplex (predominantly type 1), lymphocytic choriomeningitis, mumps, post-infectious (following influenza, measles, mumps, rubella, varicella-zoster), rabies. Post-vaccination: Rabies, pertussis.	CSF for pressure (elevated), cell count (WBCs elevated but variable [10–2000/μL], mostly lymphocytes), protein (elevated, especially IgG fraction), glucose (normal), RBCs (especially in herpesvirus). Repeat exam of CSF after 24 hours often useful. (See CSF profiles, p 228.) CSF cultures for virus (low yield for herpes) and bacteria (low yield). Throat swab for enterovirus, mumps. Stool culture for enterovirus, which is frequently shed for weeks (especially in children). Urine culture for mumps. Culture of both skin biopsy from hairline and saliva for rabies. Histologic examination of brain biopsy for definitive diagnosis of herpes simplex. Paired sera for arboviruses, mumps, or rabies should be drawn acutely and after 1–3 weeks of illness. Serologic tests are often of academic interest only. Not indicated for herpes simplex.	Herpes simplex: High-dose acyclovir. Other causes: Supportive care.	Controversy exists over whether brain biopsy is necessary for diagnosis and treatment of herpes simplex. CT scan with contrast or MRI with gadolinium reveals temporal lobe lesions consistent with herpes simplex. Ref: Pediatr Infect Dis J 1987;6:2. Ref: Rev Infect Dis 1984; 6:608.

CENTRAL NERVOUS SYSTEM			
Aseptic Meningitis			
Aseptic Meningitis	CSF for pressure (elevated), cell count (WBCs 10–100/μL, PMNs early, lymphocytes later), protein (normal or slightly elevated), and glucose (normal). (See CSF profiles, p 228.)	Most cases: Supportive care. Broad-spectrum antibiotics may be prudent in first few days of severe or atypical infection (see Bacterial meningitis, below).	Aseptic meningitis is acute meningeal irritation in the absence of pyogenic bacteria or fungi. Diagnosis is usually made by the examination of the CSF and by ruling out other infectious causes (eg, syphilis, tuberculosis).
Enteroviruses (coxsackie, echo, polio) (90%), mumps, herpes simplex (HSV, predominantly type 2), varicella-zoster (VZV), leptospirosis (rare).	CSF viral culture can be negative despite active viral infection. Enteroviruses can be isolated from the CSF in the first few days after onset but only rarely after the first week.		Enteroviral aseptic meningitis is rare after age 40. Ref: Am J Epidemiol 1969; 89:51.
	Stool culture for viral identification, especially enterovirus.		
	Throat swab or nasopharyngeal washing (in children) for enterovirus, mumps.		
	Urine viral culture for mumps.		
	Vesicle culture for HSV or VZV.		
	Paired sera for viral titers: poliovirus, mumps, and VZV. Not practical for other organisms unless actual isolate known and then only useful epidemiologically.		
	Blood or urine for serologic test for leptospirosis (very expensive; should be ordered only with very high index of suspicion).		
	Vesicle fluid for direct fluorescent antibody testing for HSV or VZV.		

	CENTRAL NERVOUS SYSTEM		
	Bacterial Meningitis		
Organism	**Specimens/Diagnostic Tests**	**Therapy**	**Comments**
Bacterial Meningitis Neonate: *E coli* (GNR), group B or D streptococci (GPC). Infant: Group B or D streptococci, *H influenzae* (GNCB). *S pneumoniae* (GPC), *N meningitidis* (GNDC), *Listeria monocytogenes* (GPR). Child: *H influenzae*, *S pneumoniae*, *N meningitidis*. Adult: *S pneumoniae*, *N meningitidis*, *Listeria*. Post-neurosurgical: *S aureus* (GPC), *S pneumoniae*, *Pseudomonas* (GNR), *E coli* (GNR), other Enterobacteriaceae. Alcoholic patients and the elderly: Enterobacteriaceae, *Pseudomonas*, *H influenzae*.	CSF for pressure (> 180 mm H$_2$O), cell count (WBCs 1000–100,000/µL, > 50% PMNs), protein (150–500 mg/dL), glucose (< 40% of serum). (See CSF profiles, p 228.) CSF sediment for Gram's stain (positive in 70–80%). CSF culture for bacteria. Blood culture positive in 40–60% of patients with pneumococcal, meningococcal, and *H influenzae* meningitis. CSF CIE or latex agglutination antigen test may be useful for rapid detection of pneumococcus, *H influenzae* type B capsular polysaccharide, group B *Streptococcus*, or meningococcus when smear and culture fail to make diagnosis. False-negative results are common. Antigen tests on concentrated urine may be more sensitive in systemic infection but are not necessarily indicative of CSF infection.	Infant: IV AMP + IV Ceph 3.* Child: IV Ceph 3 or cefuroxime + dexamethasone.* Adult: HD Pen G or IV Ceph 3. If *Listeria* is suspected, add IV AMP.* Post-neurosurgical: Vanc + ceftizoxime.* In infants and children, 7 days of therapy adequate for *H influenzae*, *S pneumoniae*, meningococcus; 10 days for group B streptococcus; 21 days for Enterobacteriaceae. In general, treatment should be continued for 10 days if CSF shows WBCs > 200/µL, glucose < 30 mg/dL, or protein > 200 mg/dL at 7 days.*	The first priority in the care of the patient with suspected acute meningitis is therapy, then diagnosis. Antibiotics should be started within 30 minutes of presentation. The death rate for meningitis is about 30%. Dexamethasone therapy for the first 4 days has been reported to decrease the risk of deafness in children with meningitis. The use of dexamethasone in adults is still under study, but many recommend using 12 mg IV q12h × 3 days. Ref: Pediatr Infect Dis J 1987;6:501. Ref: N Engl J Med 1988; 319: 964. Ref: Pediatr Infect Dis J 1989;8: 848.

*Adapted and reproduced, with permission, from Sanford JP: *Guide to Antimicrobial Therapy 1991*, Antimicrobial Therapy, Inc, 1991.

CENTRAL NERVOUS SYSTEM		
Fungal Meningitis		
Fungal Meningitis *Cryptococcus neoformans* (spherical, budding yeast), *Coccidioides immitis* (spherules), *Histoplasma capsulatum*.	CSF for pressure (normal or elevated), cell count (WBCs 50–1000/μL, mostly lymphocytes), protein (elevated), and glucose (decreased). CSF for fungal culture (collect at least 5 mL). Initial cultures are positive in 75% of cases of cryptococcal meningitis, 40% of *Coccidioides* cases. Repeat cultures are frequently needed. Culture of blood and sputum for fungus should also be performed to rule out extraneural infection. CSF India ink prep for *Cryptococcus* is not recommended because it is positive in only 50% of cases. CSF cryptococcal antigen (CrAg) is a latex agglutination test. It is positive in 95% of AIDS cases, 85% of non-AIDS patients with cryptococcal meningitis. Serum CrAg is positive in 98% of AIDS patients with cryptococcal meningitis. Serum coccidioidal serology is a concentrated serum immunodiffusion test for the organism (75–95%). CSF serology rarely necessary. (See Coccidioidal serology, p 66.) Complement fixation test for *Histoplasma* is available from Public Health Labs (see p 93).	Ampho (± 5FC) for primary therapy. Low-dose Ampho or fluconazole for prevention of relapses in immunocompromised and AIDS patients.	The clinical presentation of fungal meningitis is that of an indolent chronic meningitis. Prior to AIDS, cryptococcal meningitis was seen both in patients with cellular immunologic deficiencies and in patients who lacked obvious defects (about 50% of cases). *Cryptococcus* is the most common cause of meningitis in AIDS patients. HIV-related cryptococcal meningitis may present with totally normal CSF findings. In AIDS patients, the use of 5FC with Ampho is not supported by all studies. Some studies have shown no improvement in outcome with increased toxicity. Ref: N Engl J Med 1989; 321:794.

		CENTRAL NERVOUS SYSTEM	
		Spirochetal Meningitis	**Tuberculous Meningitis**
Organism			
Spirochetal Meningitis/ Neurosyphilis *Treponema pallidum*	**Specimens/Diagnostic Tests**	**Acute syphilitic meningitis:** CSF for pressure (elevated), cell count (WBCs 25–2000/μL, mostly lymphocytes), protein (elevated), and glucose (normal or low). (See CSF profiles, p 228.) Serum VDRL. (See Table, serum, p 138.) CSF VDRL is the preferred test (see p 139), but is only 66% sensitive for acute syphilitic meningitis. **Neurosyphilis:** CSF for pressure (normal), cell count (WBCs normal or slightly increased, mostly lymphocytes), protein (normal or elevated), and glucose (normal). Serum VDRL, FTA-ABS or MHA-TP, and CSF VDRL should also be done.	
	Therapy	HD Pen. Desensitization may be required if patient is Pen allergic. Therapy of suspected neurosyphilis should not be withheld on the basis of a negative CSF VDRL if clinical suspicion is high.	
	Comments	Neurosyphilis is a late stage of infection and can present with meningovascular (hemiparesis, seizures, aphasia), parenchymal (general paresis), tabes dorsalis), or asymptomatic (latent) disease. Neurosyphilis often has an accelerated atypical presentation in HIV-infected patients and often recurs after therapy. Serologic tests are less reliable. Ref: JAMA 1981;246:2613.	
Tuberculous Meningitis *Mycobacterium tuberculosis* (MTb) (acid-fast bacilli [AFB] seen on Kinyoun stain)			CSF for pressure (elevated), cell count (WBCs 100–500/μL, PMNs early, lymphocytes later), protein (elevated), glucose (decreased). (See CSF profiles, p 228.) CSF for AFB stain (see Kinyoun stain, p 27). Stain is positive in only 30%. CSF for AFB culture (positive in < 70%). Repeated sampling of the CSF during the first week of therapy is recommended; ideally, 3–4 specimens of 5–10 mL each should be obtained (87% yield with 4 specimens). Standard cultures for MTb take 6–8 weeks to turn positive. A new radiometric culture system (Bactec) may detect mycobacterial growth in several days.
			6-month protocol: INH, Rif, PZA, EMB for 2 months; INH, Rif for remaining 4 months (if sensitivities show mycobacteria sensitive to INH and Rif). Many recommend corticosteroid therapy for patients with focal neurologic deficits or altered mental status.
			Tuberculous meningitis is usually secondary to rupture of a subependymal tubercle rather than blood-borne invasion. Since CSF stain and culture are not sensitive for tuberculosis, diagnosis and treatment should be based on a combination of clinical and microbiologic data. Evidence of inactive or active extrameningeal tuberculosis, especially pulmonary, is seen in 75% of patients.

	CNS	EYE
	Subdural Empyema	**Conjunctivitis**

Subdural Empyema		
Infant and Child: Group B or D streptococci (GPC), *H influenzae* (GNCB), *S pneumoniae* (GPC), *N meningitidis* (GNDC). Adult: Usually polymicrobial: Viridans group streptococci (GPC in chains) (35%), *S aureus* (GPC) (17%), anaerobic streptococci (GPC in chains) (12%), *Bacteroides* (GPR), Enterobacteriaceae (GNR).	At least 2 mL of CSF should be sent to the lab immediately for culture. Since anaerobic cultures have a yield of less than 1%, they are not routinely performed and must be requested if clinical suspicion exists. Latex particle agglutination test for rapid detection of pneumococcal and meningococcal antigen can speed diagnosis. Since subdural empyemas are uncommon, most antigen testing done is negative.	Infant: IV AMP + IV Ceph 3. Child: IV Ceph 3 or cefuroxime. Adult: Nafcillin + Metr or Vanc + Metr.	Subdural empyema usually occurs as an extension of paranasal sinus infection, osteomyelitis of the skull with epidural abscess, or middle ear or mastoid infection. Sinusitis or otitis is present on skull x-rays or CT scans in over two-thirds of patients. If CT is negative, angiography is helpful.
Conjunctivitis			
Neonate (ophthalmia neonatorum): *N gonorrhoeae* (GNDC), *Chlamydia trachomatis*, herpes simplex type 2. Adult: Adenovirus, *H influenzae* (GNCB), *S pneumoniae* (GPC), group A streptococcus (GPC), *N gonorrhoeae* (GNDC), *Moraxella lacunata*. Acute hemorrhagic conjunctivitis (acute epidemic keratoconjunctivitis): Enterovirus, coxsackievirus. Adult inclusion conjunctivitis/ Trachoma: *Chlamydia trachomatis*.	Conjunctival Gram's stain is especially useful if gonococcal infection suspected. Bacterial culture for severe cases (routine bacterial culture) or suspected gonococcal infection (chocolate agar). Conjunctival scrapings or smears for *Chlamydia* show epithelial intracytoplasmic inclusions by Giemsa stain (10–60% sensitivity). Cell culture for *Chlamydia*.	Neonate: Treat according to suspected agent (see below). Adult: Topical neomycin-polymyxin or sulfonamide ointment for bacterial causes. Acute hemorrhagic conjunctivitis: None. Adult inclusion conjunctivitis/ Trachoma: Tcn or Eryth for minimum of 3 weeks. Treat sexual partners. Gonococcal: IV Pen G or cefotaxime with topical treatment and frequent saline lavage.	The causes of conjunctivitis change with the season. Adenovirus occurs mainly in the fall, *H influenzae* in the winter. Gonococcal conjunctivitis is an ophthalmologic emergency. Cultures are usually unnecessary unless *Chlamydia* or gonorrhea is suspected, or the case is severe. Ref: Surv Ophthalmol 1987;32:199. Ref: Ophthalmology 1986; 93: 456.

	EYE		
	Keratitis		**Endophthalmitis**
Organism	**Specimens/Diagnostic Tests**	**Therapy**	**Comments**
Keratitis Bacteria: *Pseudomonas aeruginosa* (GNR), *S pneumoniae* (GPDC), *Moraxella* sp, *Staphylococcus* sp (GPC). Virus: Herpes simplex (HSV) (dendritic pattern on fluorescein slitlamp exam) Contact lens: *Acanthamoeba.* Fungus: *Candida.*	Corneal scrapings for Gram's stain and culture (bring to lab promptly). Routine bacterial culture is used for most bacterial causes, viral culture for herpes, and special media for *Acanthamoeba* (can be detected with trichrome or Giemsa stain of smears). Treatment depends on Gram's stain appearance and culture.	GPC: Topical, subconjunctival, and IV cefazolin. GNR: Topical, subconjunctival, and IV tobramycin. No organisms: Topical, subconjunctival Ceph 1 + tobramycin and IV TC/CL. Virus (HSV): Topical trifluridine. Contact lens: Neomycin-polymyxin B-gramicidin + propamidine + clotrimazole cream. Fungus: Topical pimaricin, subconjunctival miconazole.	Prompt ophthalmologic consultation is mandatory. *Acanthamoeba* may resemble HSV on fluorescein examination (dendritic "branching" ulcer). Ref: Arch Ophthalmology 1986; 104:1287. Ref: Arch Ophthalmology 1988; 106:1196. Ref: Am J Ophthalmology 1986; 102:527.
Endophthalmitis Spontaneous or postoperative: *S aureus* (GPC), *S epidermidis* (GPC), Enterobacteriaceae (GNR), *Pseudomonas* sp (GNR), anaerobes, fungus (especially in neutropenic or critically ill patients). Post-filtering bleb: Viridans group streptococcus (57%), *S pneumoniae* (GPDC), *H influenzae* (GNCB). IV drug abuse: Add *B cereus* to above.	Culture material from anterior chamber, vitreous cavity, and wound abscess. Traumatic and postoperative cases should have aqueous and vitreous aspiration for culture and smear (56%). Conjunctival cultures are inadequate and misleading.	Spontaneous or postoperative: Intravitreal and IV Vanc + APAG and periocular cefotaxime + gentamicin. Post-filtering bleb: Intravitreal Vanc + APAG and periocular cefotaxime + gentamicin and IV AM/SB or Ceph 2. IV drug abuse: Add IV Clinda. Probenecid 0.5 g PO qid prolongs the half-life of beta-lactam therapy.	Endophthalmitis is an inflammatory process of the ocular cavity and adjacent structures. Bacterial endophthalmitis usually occurs as a consequence of ocular surgery. Prophylactic antibiotic use is of unproved benefit, though topical antibiotics are widely used. Ref: Am J Ophthalmology 1976;81:52.

EAR			
Otitis Media			
Otitis Media Infant, Child, and Adult: *S pneumoniae* (GPC), *H influenzae* (GNCB), *M catarrhalis* (GNDC), *S aureus* (GPC), group A *Streptococcus* (GPC), "sterile." Neonate: Same as above plus Enterobacteriaceae (GNR), group B *Streptococcus* (GPC). Endotracheal intubation: *Pseudomonas* sp (GNR), *Klebsiella* (GNR), Enterobacteriaceae (GNR).	Tympanocentesis aspirate for Gram's stain and bacterial culture in the patient who has a toxic appearance. Otherwise, microbiologic studies of effusions are so consistent that empiric treatment is acceptable. Blood culture (aerobic or anaerobic) in the toxic patient.	< 4 years old: Eryth + sulfonamide. > 4 years old: TMP/SMX or AMP/X. Endotracheal intubation: IV ceftazidime or TC/CL or Aztr. Tympanocentesis is indicated if the patient fails to improve after 48 hours or develops fever. It may hasten resolution and decrease sterile effusion.	Peak incidence of otitis media occurs in the first 3 years of life, especially between 6 and 24 months of age. In neonates, predisposing factors include cleft palate, hypotonia, mental retardation (Down's syndrome). About one-third of nasotracheally intubated patients will develop otitis media with effusion after 48 hours. Ref: Pediatr Infect Dis J 1988;7(Suppl 11):S129.
Otitis Externa			
Otitis Externa Acute localized: *S aureus* (GPC), group A *Streptococcus* (GPC in chains). "Swimmer's ear": *Pseudomonas* sp (GNR), Enterobacteriaceae (GNR), fungi (rare). Chronic: Usually secondary to seborrhea. Diabetes mellitus ("malignant otitis externa"): *Pseudomonas* sp. Furuncle of external canal: *S aureus*.	Ear drainage for Gram's stain and bacterial culture, especially in malignant otitis externa.	Acute localized: Dicloxacillin or PO Ceph 1. "Swimmer's ear": Polymyxin B + neomycin + hydrocortisone eardrops qid (Cortisporin). Chronic: Polymyxin B + neomycin + hydrocortisone. Diabetes mellitus: APPen + APAG or ceftazidime + APAG. Furuncle of external canal: Incision and drainage. PO Ceph 1 or Clinda if cellulitis present.	Infection of the external auditory canal is similar to infection of skin and soft tissue elsewhere. If malignant otitis externa is present, exclusion of associated osteomyelitis and surgical drainage may be required. Ref: Am J Med 1988;85:391.

SINUS

Sinusitis

Organism	Specimens/Diagnostic Tests	Therapy	Comments
Sinusitis	Nasal aspirate for bacterial culture is not usually helpful. Maxillary sinus aspirate for bacterial culture may be helpful in severe or atypical cases.	Acute: TMP/SMX or AMP/X or AM/CL. Chronic (Child): Same as above or Eryth + sulfonamide. Chronic (Adult): HD Pen is the treatment of choice though antibiotics are usually not effective. Hospitalized with nasogastric tube or nasotracheal intubation: Ceftazidime or PRPen + APAG. Surgical drainage of sinus may be necessary in severe or refractory cases.	Diagnosis and treatment of sinusitis is usually based on clinical and radiologic features. Microbiologic studies can be helpful in severe or atypical cases. Sinus CT scan is better than plain x-ray for diagnosing sinusitis, particularly if sphenoid sinusitis is suspected. Ref: N Engl J Med 1981; 304:749.
Acute: *S pneumoniae* (GPC) (31%), *H influenzae* (GNCB) (21%), *M catarrhalis* (GNDC), group A *Streptococcus* (GPC), anaerobes, viruses (rhinovirus, influenza, parainfluenza), *S aureus* (GPC) (rare). Chronic (Child): *S pneumoniae*, *H influenzae*, *M catarrhalis*. Chronic (Adult): *Bacteroides* sp, *Peptostreptococcus* (GPC), *Fusobacterium* sp. Hospitalized with nasogastric tube or nasotracheal intubation: Enterobacteriaceae (GNR), *Pseudomonas* sp (GNR). Fungal: Zygomycetes (*Mucor*), *Aspergillus*, *Pseudallescheria boydii*.			

UPPER AIRWAY			
Pharyngitis			**Laryngitis**
Pharyngitis Exudative: Group A *Streptococcus* (GPC) (15–30%), viruses (rhinovirus, coronavirus, adenovirus) (25%), group C *Streptococcus* (GPC), Epstein-Barr virus (mononucleosis), *N gonorrhoeae* (GNDC), *Arcanobacterium* (*Corynebacterium*) *hemolyticum*. Membranous: *C diphtheriae* (GPR), Epstein-Barr virus.	Throat swab for culture. Place in sterile tube or transport medium. If *N gonorrhoeae* suspected, use chocolate agar or Thayer-Martin media. If *C diphtheriae* suspected, use Tinsdale or blood agar. Throat swabs are routinely only cultured for group A *Streptococcus*. If other organisms are suspected, this must be stated. Throat culture is about 70% sensitive for group A *Streptococcus*. "Rapid" tests (Directogen, Culturette, many others) for group A *Streptococcus* can speed diagnosis and aid in the treatment of family members. Latex agglutination systems are more specific (95–99%) for streptococcal infection than throat culture, though not as sensitive (70–90%). Solid phase ELISA tests have similar results.	Child and Adult: Pen or Eryth. *N gonorrhoeae*: Ceftriaxone IM. Asymptomatic carrier in family with case of rheumatic fever: Pen + Rif. Diphtheria: diphtheria antitoxin plus Pen or Eryth. IM benzathine Pen is preferable when compliance is questionable. Amantadine may be considered during epidemic of type A influenza.	Controversy exists over how to evaluate patients with sore throat. Some authors suggest culturing all patients and then treating only those with positive cultures. In patients with compatible histories, be sure to consider pharyngeal abscess or epiglottitis, both of which may be life-threatening. Ref: Ann Intern Med 1986; 105:892.
Laryngitis Virus (90%), group A *Streptococcus* (GPC) (10%), *Moraxella catarrhalis* (55% of adults).	Diagnosis is made by clinical picture of upper respiratory infection with hoarseness.	Antibiotics usually not indicated. Rest voice until hoarseness improves.	Laryngitis usually occurs in association with common cold or influenzal syndromes. Ref: Scand J Infect Dis 1980;12:277.

		Specimens/Diagnostic Tests	Therapy	Comments
		UPPER AIRWAY		
		Tracheobronchitis		*Epiglottitis*
Organism				
Tracheobronchitis		Throat swab or nasopharyngeal aspirate for viral, *Mycoplasma* or *Bordetella* culture can be considered in acute cases (rarely indicated). Cellular exam of early morning sputum will show many PMNs in chronic bronchitis.	Infant/Child: Aerosolized ribavirin if child is sick enough to be hospitalized. Otherwise, no treatment is indicated.	Chronic bronchitis by definition is diagnosed when sputum is coughed up on most days for at least 3 consecutive months for more than 2 successive years.
Infant/Child (Bronchiolitis): Respiratory syncytial virus (50–75%), parainfluenza virus, adenovirus.			Adolescent/Adult: None indicated. If infiltrate is present on chest x-ray, treat as primary pneumonia with Eryth or Tcn.	Bacterial infections are usually secondary infections of initial viral or *Mycoplasma*-induced inflammation.
Adolescent/Adult: Usually viruses, *Mycoplasma pneumoniae, Chlamydia pneumoniae, Bordetella pertussis.*		Sputum Gram's stain and culture for ill adults. In chronic bronchitis, mixed flora are usually seen with oral flora or colonized *H influenzae* or *S pneumoniae* on culture.	Chronic: TMP/SMX or Tcn or AM/CL.	
Chronic adult (smokers): Viral (25–50%), *S pneumoniae* (GPC), *H influenzae* (GNCB), *S aureus* (GPC), Enterobacteriaceae (GNR), anaerobes (< 10%).		Paired sera for viral titers can help make a diagnosis retrospectively but are not clinically useful except for seriously ill patients.	In exacerbations of chronic bronchitis, corticosteroids may shorten course.	
Epiglottitis		Blood for bacterial culture: positive in 50–100% of children with *H influenzae*.	Child or Adult: IV Ceph 3 or Ceph 2 or chloramphenicol.	Acute epiglottitis is a rapidly moving cellulitis of the epiglottis and represents an airway emergency.
Child: *H influenzae* type B (GNCB).		Throat/epiglottis swab for Gram's stain and bacterial culture can be helpful in adults but is not indicated in children because it can precipitate laryngospasm and acute airway obstruction.	Dexamethasone may lessen the severity and shorten the course of disease.	Epiglottitis can be confused with croup, a viral infection of gradual onset that affects infants and causes inspiratory and expiratory stridor.
Adult: Group A *Streptococcus* (GPC), *H influenzae.*		Lateral neck x-ray may show an enlarged epiglottis but has a low sensitivity (31%).	Airway management is the primary concern, and endotracheal tube or tracheostomy should be placed as soon as diagnosis is made in children. A tracheostomy set should be at the bedside for adults.	Ref: Crit Care Med 1986; 14:23.

LUNG			
Community-Acquired Pneumonia			
Community-Acquired Pneumonia Neonate: *E coli* (GNR), group A or B *Streptococcus* (GPC), *S aureus* (GPC), *Pseudomonas* sp (GNR), *Chlamydia trachomatis*. Infant/Child (< 5 years): Virus, *S pneumoniae* (GPC), *H influenzae* (GNCB), *S aureus*. Age 5–40 years: Virus, *Mycoplasma pneumoniae*, *Chlamydia pneumoniae* and *C psittaci*, *S pneumoniae*, *Legionella* sp. Age > 40 without other disease: *S pneumoniae*, group A *Streptococcus*, *H influenzae*, *Legionella* sp, *Chlamydia pneumoniae* (TWAR strain), *C psittaci*, viruses (eg, influenza). Chronic bronchitis: *S pneumoniae*, group A streptococcus, *H influenzae*, *Klebsiella* (GNR), other Enterobacteriaceae (GNR), virus (eg, influenza). Underlying disease (alcoholism, diabetes, CHF): As in chronic bronchitis with addition of *M pneumoniae*, *Legionella* sp, *C pneumoniae*, *S aureus*. Cystic fibrosis: *Pseudomonas aeruginosa*, *P cepacia*.	Sputum for Gram's stain and culture. An adequate specimen should have < 10 epithelial cells and > 25 PMNs per low-power field. Special sputum cultures for *C trachomatis*, TWAR, and *Legionella* are available. Blood for bacterial cultures, especially in ill patients. Pleural fluid for bacterial culture if significant effusion is present. Bronchoalveolar lavage or brushings for bacterial, fungal, and AFB culture in immunocompromised patients and atypical cases. Paired sera for *M pneumoniae* complement fixation testing can diagnose infection retrospectively. Serologic tests for *C pneumoniae* (including TWAR) and *C psittaci* strains are available.	Neonate: IV AMP + AG or PRPen + AG.* Infant/Child (< 5 years): Usually none. PRPen + APAG, if serious life-threatening infection.* Age 5–40 years: Eryth or doxycycline or LD Pen if pneumococcus by Gram's stain.* Age > 40: Ceph 3 or cefuroxime. Chronic bronchitis: Ceph 3 or TC/CL.* Underlying disease (alcoholism, diabetes, CHF): Eryth + Ceph 3 or cefuroxime or TMP/SMX.* Cystic fibrosis: Tobramycin + APPen or Ceph 3 or Aztr. If *P cepacia*, then TMP/SMX.* In infants and children, IV therapy should be continued until the patient is afebrile for 72–96 hours.* In adults, if sputum Gram's stain shows pneumococcus, Pen G intravenously alone is sufficient.*	About 60% of cases of community-acquired pneumonia have an identifiable microbial etiology. Pneumatoceles suggest *S aureus* but are also reported with pneumococcus, group A *Streptococcus*, *H influenzae*, and Enterobacteriaceae (ie neonates). An "atypical pneumonia" presentation (diffuse pattern on chest x-ray with lack of organisms on Gram's stain of sputum) should raise suspicion of *Mycoplasma*, *Legionella*, or chlamydial infection and warrants empiric treatment with Eryth. During type A influenza epidemics, amantadine may shorten course of disease if given in the first 1–2 days of illness. Ref: Chest 1988;94:1076. Ref: Medicine 1990;69:307.

* Adapted and reproduced, with permission, from Sanford JP: *Guide to Antimicrobial Therapy 1991*, Antimicrobial Therapy, Inc, 1991.

	Organism	Specimens/Diagnostic Tests	Therapy	Comments
LUNG				
Anaerobic Pneumonia/Lung Abscess	Usually polymicrobial: *Bacteroides* sp (15% *B fragilis*), *Peptostreptococcus, Fusobacterium* sp, type 3 *S pneumoniae* (rare), *Klebsiella* (rare).	Sputum Gram's stain and culture for anaerobes are usually of little value because of contaminating oral flora. Bronchoalveolar sampling (brush or aspirate) for bacterial culture will usually make an accurate diagnosis. As contamination is likely with a bronchoscope alone, a Bartlett tube should be used. Percutaneous transthoracic needle aspiration may be useful for culture but provides small or less adequate samples. Blood cultures are usually negative.	Clinda or HD Pen G.* Metr is not as effective as Clinda in putrid lung abscess.*	Aspiration is the most important background feature of lung abscess. Without clear-cut risk factors such as alcoholism, coma, or seizures, bronchoscopy is often performed to rule out neoplasm. Ref: Chest 1987;91:901
Aspiration Pneumonia	Community-acquired: *S pneumoniae* (GPC), *Klebsiella pneumoniae* (GNR), Enterobacteriaceae (GNR), *Bacteroides* sp and other oral anaerobes. Hospital-associated: *Pseudomonas* sp (GNR), *Klebsiella*. Neutropenic: *Pseudomonas* sp (GNR), *Klebsiella, Enterobacter* (GNR), *Bacteroides* sp and other oral anaerobes, *Legionella, Candida, Aspergillus, Mucor.* Mendelson's syndrome (see comments): No organisms initially, then *Pseudomonas,* Enterobacteriaceae, *S aureus, S pneumoniae.*	Sputum Gram's stain and culture for bacteria (aerobic and anaerobic) and fungus (if suspected). Blood cultures for bacteria are often negative. Endotracheal aspirate or bronchoalveolar sample for bacterial and fungal culture in selected patients.	Community-acquired: Clinda + AG or cefoxitin.* Hospital-associated (associated with intubation, broad-spectrum antibiotics): APPen + APAG or Ceph 3 + APAG or IMP. If GPC on Gram's stain, add PRPen or Vanc.* Neutropenic: Vanc + APAG + APPen or ceftazidime or IMP + APAG + Eryth. If bronchoscopy positive for *Legionella* or fungal elements, add Eryth or Ampho.* Mendelson's syndrome: None or LD Pen G.*	Community-acquired aspirations are most commonly associated with stroke, alcoholism, drug abuse, and sedation. Hospital-associated aspiration pneumonia is associated with intubation and the use of broad-spectrum antibiotics. Mendelson's syndrome is due to acute aspiration of gastric contents (eg, during anesthesia or drowning).

*Adapted and reproduced, with permission, from Sanford JP: *Guide to Antimicrobial Therapy 1991*, Antimicrobial Therapy, Inc, 1991.

LUNG		
Pneumonia in AIDS		
Pneumonia in the HIV-Infected Host Child: Lymphoid interstitial pneumonia (LIP). Adult: *Pneumocystis carinii* (PCP), *S pneumoniae* (GPC), *H influenzae* (GNCB), *M tuberculosis* (AFB), *Histoplasma, Coccidioides, Cryptococcus*.	Expectorated sputum for Gram's stain and bacterial culture, if purulent. Sputum induction for Giemsa or methenamine silver staining or direct fluorescent antibody (DFA) for *Pneumocystis carinii* trophozoites or cysts; and for mycobacterial and fungal staining and culture. Blood or bone marrow fungal culture for histoplasmosis (positive in 50%), coccidioidomycosis (positive in 30%). Blood culture for bacteria (aerobic and anaerobic). Blood cultures are more frequently positive in HIV-infected patients with pneumococcal pneumonia and often are the only source where a specific organism is identified. *Histoplasma* polysaccharide antigen: positive in 90% of AIDS patients with disseminated histoplasmosis. Immunodiffusion or CIE is useful for screening for and CF for confirmation of suspected histoplasmosis or coccidioidomycosis. Cryptococcal antigen serology when pulmonary cryptococcosis is suspected.	Child: Corticosteroids. Suspected bacterial pneumonia: See Community-acquired pneumonia. Suspected PCP: TMP/SMX, pentamidine. Second line: TMP/dapsone or Clinda/primaquine (after testing for G6PD deficiency). Fungal pneumonia: Ampho B. Ketoconazole for prevention of relapses. Itraconazole is a promising new agent for therapy and prophylaxis.	In PCP the sensitivities of the various diagnostic tests are: sputum induction 80% (in experienced labs), bronchoscopy with lavage 90–97%, transbronchial biopsy 94–97%. PCP prophylaxis is recommended for all HIV-infected adults after a first episode of PCP or with CD4 cells < 200/µL. Preferred prophylactic agent is TMP/SMX. Other effective agents include inhaled pentamidine and dapsone. Kaposi's sarcoma of the lung is a common neoplastic process that can imitate infection in homosexual and African HIV-infected patients. Ref: Am J Med 1989;87: 396. Ref: Med Clin North Am 1988;72(5):1067.

	LUNG		
	Mycobacterial Pneumonia		
Organism	Specimens/Diagnostic Tests	Therapy	Comments
Mycobacterial Pneumonia *Mycobacterium tuberculosis* (MTb), *M kansasii*, *M avium-intracellulare* complex (AFB, acid-fast beaded rods)	Sputum for AFB stain and culture. First morning samples are best, and at least 3 samples are required. Standard cultures for MTb take 6–8 weeks to turn positive. A new radiometric culture system (Bactec) may detect mycobacterial growth in as little as several days. Bronchoalveolar lavage for AFB stain and culture or gastric washings for AFB culture can be used if sputum tests are negative.	6-month regimen: INH, Rif, PZA, EMB for 2 months, then INH, Rif for remaining 4 months (if MTb sensitive to these agents). Antibiotic-resistant (especially INH-resistant) organisms require more aggressive therapy. Persons with a positive PPD and negative sputum smear and CXR should receive INH prophylaxis if they are under 21 years old, a recent converter, HIV-infected, or have recent exposure to a household contact with active MTb. Treatment of nontuberculous mycobacteria is complicated and depends on organism sensitivities.	AFB found on sputum stain does not necessarily make the diagnosis of tuberculosis, because *M kansasii* and *M avium-intracellulare* look identical. Tuberculosis is very common in HIV-infected patients, and treatment is similar to that in normal hosts. Chest x-ray appearance of MTb may be atypical in HIV-infected patients and may mimic PCP (especially in patients with CD4 cell counts < 200/μL). In any patient with suspected tuberculosis, respiratory isolation is required. Ref: Ann Intern Med 1987; 106:254.

	LUNG		HEART AND VESSELS
	Empyema		**Pericarditis**
Empyema Neonate: *E coli* (GNR), group A or B *Streptococcus* (GPC), *S aureus* (GPC), *Pseudomonas* sp (GNR). Infant/Child (< 5 years): *S aureus*, *S pneumoniae* (GPC), *H influenzae* (GNCB). Child (> 5 years)/Adult, Acute: *S pneumoniae*, group A *Streptococcus*, *H influenzae*, *Legionella*. Child (> 5 years)/Adult, Chronic: Anaerobic streptococci, *Bacteroides* sp, Enterobacteriaceae.	Pleural fluid for cell count (WBCs 25,000–100,000/μL, mostly PMNs), protein (> 50% of serum), glucose (< serum, often very low), pH (<7.20), LDH (> 60% of serum). (See Pleural fluid profiles, p 232.) Pleural fluid for Gram's stain and bacterial culture (aerobic and anaerobic). Blood cultures for bacteria (aerobic and anaerobic). Sputum for Gram's stain and bacterial culture. Special culture can also be performed for *Legionella* when suspected. Pleural fluid for bacterial antigens by CIE or latex agglutination can be sent if diagnosis is in question. Fluid can also be tested for *Legionella* by direct fluorescent antibody.	Chest tube drainage is para-mount. Neonate: IV AMP + AG or PRPen + AG. Infant/Child (< 5 years): PRPen + APAG. In adults, if organisms are not seen: Clinda + APAG or cefoxitin or Ceph 3 or TC/CL or AM/SB. If *S pneumoniae*/group A *Streptococcus*: HD Pen G. If *S aureus*: PRPen. If *H influenzae*: Ceph 3.	The clinical presentation of empyema is nonspecific, and diagnosis requires a high index of suspicion. Chest CT with contrast is helpful in demonstrating pleural fluid accumulations due to mediastinal or sub-diaphragmatic processes and can identify loculated effusions, bronchopleural fistulae, and lung abscesses. Ref: Am Rev Respir Dis 1987;136:1030.
Pericarditis Viruses: Enteroviruses (coxsackie, echo), influenza, Epstein-Barr, herpes zoster, mumps, HIV. Bacteria: *S aureus* (GPC), group A *Streptococcus* (GPC), Enterobacteriaceae (GNR), *N meningitidis* (GNDC).	In acute pericarditis, specific bacterial diagnosis is made in only 19%. Pericardial fluid aspirate for viral culture (rarely positive) and Gram's stain and bacterial culture (aerobic and anaerobic). In acute pericarditis, only 54% have pericardial effusions. Stool or throat swab for viral culture (if enteroviruses suspected). Surgical pericardial drainage with biopsy of pericardium for culture (22%) and histologic examination. Paired sera for enteroviruses can be helpful.	Viral: Anti-inflammatory agents (aspirin or indomethacin) or corticosteroids in unresponsive cases. Bacterial: PRPen + APAG or TC/CL or AM/SB. Surgical drainage required.	Viral pericarditis is usually diagnosed clinically. The diagnosis is rarely aided by microbiologic tests. Bacterial pericarditis is usually secondary to surgery, immunosuppression, esophageal rupture, endocarditis with ruptured ring abscess, extension from lung abscess or aspiration pneumonia or sepsis with pericarditis. Ref: Am J Card 1985;56:623.

		HEART AND VESSELS	
		Tuberculous Pericarditis	**Infectious Myocarditis**

Organism	Specimens/Diagnostic Tests	Therapy	Comments
Tuberculous Pericarditis *Mycobacterium tuberculosis* (MTb, AFB, acid-fast beaded rods)	PPD skin testing should be performed (negative in a sizeable minority). Pericardial fluid obtained by needle aspiration can show AFB by smear (rare) or culture (low yield). The yield is improved by obtaining repeated specimens (3–4) for smear and culture. Pericardial biopsy may be needed to make diagnosis and initiate early drug therapy. Other sources of culture for MTb besides pericardium are available in 50% of patients.	6-month protocol: INH, Rif, PZA, EMB for 2 months; INH, Rif for remaining 4 months (if sensitivities show MTb sensitive to INH and Rif). Corticosteroids are useful early in therapy to prevent late complications (eg. constrictive pericarditis). Surgical pericardiectomy may be necessary for one-third to one-half of patients who develop constrictive pericarditis despite drug therapy.	Spread from nearby caseous mediastinal lymph nodes or pleurisy is the most common route of infection. Acutely, serofibrinous pericardial effusion develops with substernal pain, fever, and friction rub. Tamponade may occur. Tuberculosis accounts for 4% of cases of acute pericarditis, 7% of cases of cardiac tamponade, and 6% of cases of constrictive pericarditis. Constrictive pericarditis occurs 2–4 years after acute infection. Ref: JAMA 1991;266:99.
Infectious Myocarditis Enteroviruses (coxsackie, echo, polio), HIV, *Borrelia burgdorferi* (Lyme disease), scrub typhus, *Rickettsia rickettsii* (Rocky Mountain spotted fever), *Coxiella burnetii* (Q fever), *C diphtheriae*, *Trichinella spiralis* (trichinosis), *Trypanosoma cruzi* (Chagas' disease), *Toxoplasma*.	Endomyocardial biopsy for pathology and culture in selected cases. Stool or throat swab for coxsackievirus. Paired sera for enteroviruses, scrub typhus, *Rickettsia rickettsii*, *Coxiella burnetii*, *Trichinella*, *Toxoplasma*. Single serum for HIV, *Borrelia burgdorferi*, *Trypanosoma cruzi*. Gallium scanning is sensitive but not specific for myocardial inflammation.	Viral: Supportive therapy. Other: Specific antimicrobial therapy when organism is identified. Immunosuppressive therapy with corticosteroids may improve outcome when process is acute (< 6 months) and biopsy suggests acute inflammation.	The value of endomyocardial biopsy in patients presenting with acute myocarditis has not been established. Many patients with acute myocarditis progress to dilated cardiomyopathy. Ref: N Engl J Med 1985; 312:885. Ref: N Engl J Med 1991; 325:763. Ref: West J Med 1989; 150:431.

HEART AND VESSELS			
Infective Endocarditis			
Infective Endocarditis Viridans group *Streptococcus* (GPC), *Enterococcus* (GPC), nutritionally deficient *Streptococcus* (GPC), *S aureus* (GPC), *S pneumoniae* (GPC), the HACEK group of organisms (slow-growing fastidious GNRs: *H parainfluenzae*, *H aphrophilus*, *Actinobacillus*, *Cardiobacterium*, *Eikenella*, *Kingella*).	Blood cultures for bacteria (aerobic and anaerobic). Three blood cultures are sufficient in 97% of cases. Draw before or during chills or at time of temperature spike if possible. Blood cultures are frequently positive with gram-positive organisms but can be negative with gram-negative or anaerobic organisms. If the patient is not acutely ill, therapy can begin after cultures identify an organism.	Empiric: HD Pen G + gentamicin or Vanc.* Empiric if heart failure, new valvular regurgitation or associated pneumonia or meningitis: PRPen + Gentamicin or Vanc or IV Ceph 1 + gentamicin.* Viridans group *Streptococcus*: Pen G or Vanc. If patient < 65 years old and without hearing or renal impairment, add gentamicin.* *Enterococcus*, nutritionally deficient *Streptococcus*: Pen G + gentamicin or Vanc. *S aureus*: PRPen + gentamicin or IV Ceph 1 or Vanc.* HACEK: Ceph 3 + gentamicin.*	Patients with congenital or valvular heart disease should receive prophylaxis before dental procedures or surgery of the upper respiratory, genitourinary, or gastrointestinal tract. Endocarditis prophylaxis: dental/upper airway, AMP or Eryth; genitourinary/gastrointestinal, AMP + gentamicin or Vanc + gentamicin. In left-sided endocarditis, patients should be watched carefully for development of valvular regurgitation or ring abscess. Ref: Ann Intern Med 1988; 109:619.

*Adapted and reproduced, with permission, from Sanford JP: *Guide to Antimicrobial Therapy 1991*, Antimicrobial Therapy, Inc., 1991.

		HEART AND VESSELS		
		Prosthetic Valve Infective Endocarditis		
	Organism	**Specimens/Diagnostic Tests**	**Therapy**	**Comments**
	Prosthetic Valve Infective Endocarditis (PVE) Early (< 2 months): *S epidermidis* (GPC) (27%), *S aureus* (GPC) (20%), Enterobacteriaceae (GNR), diphtheroids (GPR), *Candida, Aspergillus.* Late (> 2 months): Viridans group *Streptococcus* (GPC) (42%), *S epidermidis* (21%), *S aureus* (11%), *Enterococcus* (GPC), Enterobacteriaceae.	Blood cultures for bacteria (aerobic and anaerobic). Three sets of blood cultures are sufficient in 97% of cases. Draw before temperature spike. Blood for fungal culture in suspected cases (eg, large vegetations on echocardiogram).	Early: Vanc + gentamicin + Rif (6 weeks) or PRPen or Ceph 3 + gentamicin. Add Ampho + 5FC for fungal infection. Late: Vanc + gentamicin (6 weeks). In cases of fungal infection, surgery is mandatory. Surgical intervention should be strongly considered when there is a nonstreptococcal agent, a new regurgitant murmur, or moderate to severe heart failure.	In a large series using perioperative prophylaxis the incidences of early-onset and late-onset prosthetic valve endocarditis were 0.78% and 1.1%, respectively. The portals of entry of early-onset PVE are intraoperative contamination and postoperative wound infections. The portals of entry of late-onset PVE appear to be the same as those of native valve endocarditis, and the microbiologic profiles are also similar. Clinically, patients with late-onset PVE resemble those with native valve disease. However, those with early-onset infection are often critically ill, more often have other complicating problems, are more likely to go into shock and are more likely to have conduction abnormalities due to ring abscess. Ref: Mayo Clin Proc 1982; 57:155.

HEART AND VESSELS
Infectious Thrombophlebitis

Infectious Thrombophlebitis			
Infectious Thrombophlebitis Associated with venous catheters: *S aureus* (GPC) (65–78%), *S epidermidis* (GPC), *Candida* sp, *Pseudomonas* sp (GNR), Enterobacteriaceae (GNR). Hyperalimentation with catheter: *Candida* sp. Indwelling venous catheter (eg, Broviac, Hickman, Gershorn): *S aureus*, *S epidermidis*, *Pseudomonas* sp, Enterobacteriaceae, *Candida* sp. Postpartum or post-abortion pelvic thrombophlebitis: *Bacteroides* (GNR), Enterobacteriaceae, *Clostridium* (GPR), *Streptococcus* (GPC).	Blood cultures for bacteria (aerobic and anaerobic) (positive in 80–90%). Catheter tip for bacterial culture. More than 15 colonies (CFUs) suggests colonization or infection.	Venous catheters: Vanc + Ceph 3 or Vanc + APPen. If *Candida* sp on culture or Gram's stain: Ampho. Add ketoconazole if *Candida* sensitive in vitro. Indwelling catheter: Vanc + Ceph 3 or Vanc + APPen or PRPen + APAG. Postpartum or post-abortion pelvic thrombophlebitis: Clinda + APAG or cefoxitin. Heparin is also of benefit. Treatment without removal of indwelling central venous catheters is often possible. If patient becomes septic, if bacteremia persists after 48 hours, or if significant tunnel infection is present, catheter should be removed. If fungus is isolated, catheter should be removed. If area is suppurative, surgery with venotomy is usually needed for cure.	Thrombophlebitis is an inflammation of the vein wall. Infectious thrombophlebitis is associated with microbial invasion of the vessel and is associated with bacteremia and thrombosis. Risk of infection from an indwelling peripheral venous catheter goes up significantly after 4 days. Ref: N Engl J Med 1985; 312:1142. Ref: Arch Intern Med 1987; 147: 873.

	ABDOMEN
	Infectious Esophagitis

Organism	Specimens/Diagnostic Tests	Therapy	Comments
Infectious Esophagitis			
Candida sp., herpesvirus sp (herpes simplex, cytomegalovirus, varicella-zoster), *Cryptosporidium.*	Barium esophagram reveals abnormalities in the majority of cases of candidal esophagitis. Endoscopy with biopsy and brushings for culture and cytology has the highest diagnostic yield (57%) and should be performed if clinically indicated or if empiric antifungal therapy is unsuccessful.	*Candida:* Ketoconazole, LD Ampho in poorly responsive patients. Herpes: Acyclovir. Cytomegalovirus: Ganciclovir (DHPG). *Cryptosporidium:* No treatment yet available. Spiramycin has not been effective.	Thrush and odynophagia in an immunocompromised patient warrants empiric therapy for *Candida.* Factors predisposing to infectious esophagitis include HIV infection, exposure to radiation, cytotoxic chemotherapy, recent antibiotic therapy, corticosteroid therapy, and neutropenia. Ref: Endoscopy 1987;19: 153. Ref: Rev Infect Dis 1987; 9(1): 88. Ref: Ann Intern Med 1988; 109: 471.

ABDOMEN		
Infectious Colitis/Dysentery		
Infectious Colitis/Dysentery Premature Infant (necrotizing enterocolitis): *E coli* (GNR), *S epidermidis* (GPC in clusters), *Pseudomonas aeruginosa* (GNR), *Clostridium perfringens* (GPR). Infant: *E coli* (enteropathogenic). Child/Adult without travel, afebrile, no gross blood or WBCs in stool: Rotavirus, Norwalk agent, *E coli* (GNR). Child/Adult with fever, bloody stool or WBCs in stool or history of travel to subtropics/tropics (varies with epidemiology): *Campylobacter jejuni, E coli* (enterotoxigenic, enteroinvasive, enterohemorrhagic O157:H7), *Shigella* (GNR), *Salmonella* (GNR), *Yersinia enterocolitica* (GNR), *Clostridium difficile* (GPR), *Aeromonas* (GNR), *Vibrio cholerae, Cryptosporidium, Entamoeba histolytica.*	Stool collected for stain for WBCs (Wright's or methylene blue-stained smear showing WBCs suggests invasion of the mucosa), culture, ovum and parasite examination. Multiple samples are often needed. Special culture technique is needed for *Yersinia.* Proctosigmoidoscopy is indicated in patients with chronic or recurrent diarrhea or in diarrhea of unknown cause for smears of aspirates (may show organisms) and biopsy. Rectal and jejunal biopsies may be necessary in HIV-infected patients. Use modified acid-fast stain for *Cryptosporidium.*	Premature Infant: APPen + APAG or APPen + Ceph 3. Add Vanc if *Staphylococcus* is isolated.* Infant: PO neomycin.* Child/Adult without travel, afebrile, no gross blood in stool, no WBCs in stool: None or AMP.* Child/Adult with fever, bloody stool or WBCs in stool or history of travel to subtropics/tropics (varies with epidemiology): Cipr or norfloxacin or TMP/SMX or doxycycline.* Other supportive measures can be critical. Only PO fluids or IV fluids are necessary in mild illness. Loperamide or PeptoBismol is useful in moderate illness (3–5 unformed stools/day).* In severe illness (> 6 stools/day), treat with antibiotics and IV fluid replacement (WHO solution: 4 g NaCl + 1 g KCl + 5.4 g sodium lactate + 8 g glucose/L. Volume given = fluid loss).*	Acute dysentery is diarrhea with bloody, mucoid stools, tenesmus, and pain on defecation and implies an inflammatory invasion of the colonic mucosa. Necrotizing enterocolitis is a fulminant disease of premature newborns. Air in the intestinal wall (pneumatosis intestinalis), in the portal venous system, or in the peritoneal cavity seen on plain x-ray can confirm diagnosis. 30–50% of these infants will have bacteremia or peritonitis. Ref: J Trop Med Hyg 1981; 84:73. Ref: Ann Intern Med 1972; 76: 697.

*Adapted and reproduced, with permission, from Sanford JP: *Guide to Antimicrobial Therapy 1991*, Antimicrobial Therapy, Inc, 1991.

| | ABDOMEN |
| | Antibiotic-Associated Colitis |

Organism	Specimens/Diagnostic Tests	Therapy	Comments
Antibiotic-associated/ Pseudomembranous Colitis *Clostridium difficile* (GPR) toxin.	Send stool for fecal leukocytes and *C difficile* toxin titers. Fecal WBCs are present in most cases. The toxin is very labile and can be present in patients with no disease. Stool culture using selective media can grow *C difficile* organisms, but this diagnostic method is not recommended because nontoxigenic strains occur. Colonoscopy and visualization of characteristic 1–5 mm raised yellow plaques makes the definitive diagnosis.	PO Metr or PO Vanc or PO bacitracin or cholestyramine. There is no reliable parenteral therapy. Discontinue precipitating antibiotic if possible.	Pseudomembranous colitis typically occurs after use of clindamycin, ampicillin, cephalosporins, and most other antibiotics. It may occur during drug intake or up to 2 weeks later. Other risk factors for *C difficile*-induced colitis are GI manipulations, advanced age, female sex, inflammatory bowel disease, chemotherapy, and renal disease. Ref: Am J Med 1989;86:15.

ABDOMEN
Diarrhea in HIV

Diarrhea in the HIV-infected Host			
Same as Child/Adult Infectious Colitis with addition of cytomegalovirus, *Cryptosporidium*, *Isospora belli*, microsporida, *Giardia intestinalis*, *Mycobacterium avium-intracellulare* complex, herpes simplex, *Entamoeba histolytica*. ?HIV.	Stool for stain for fecal leukocytes (Wright's or methylene blue-stained smear showing WBCs suggests invasion of the mucosa), culture (especially for *Salmonella*, *Shigella*, *Yersinia*, and *Campylobacter*), ovum and parasite examination, and AFB smear. Multiple samples are often needed. Proctosigmoidoscopy with fluid aspiration and biopsy is indicated in patients with chronic or recurrent diarrhea or in diarrhea of unknown cause for smears of aspirates (may show organisms) and histologic examination of tissue. Rectal and jejunal biopsies may be necessary, especially in patients with tenesmus or bloody stools. Use modified acid-fast stain for *Cryptosporidium*. Inclusion bodies on histologic exam suggest CMV.	Empiric therapy is not indicated. *Salmonella:* AMP or chloramphenicol. *Isospora:* TMP/SMX, pyrimethamine. Herpes: Acyclovir. Cytomegalovirus: Ganciclovir (DHPG). *Giardia:* Metr or quinacrine.	Most patients with HIV infection will develop diarrhea at some point in their illness. *Cryptosporidium* causes a chronic debilitating diarrheal infection that rarely remits spontaneously and is still without effective treatment. Diarrhea seems to be the result of malabsorption and produces a cholera-like syndrome. Ref: Infect Dis Clin North Am 1988;2(3):705. Ref: Infect Dis Clin North Am 1988;2(2):387. Ref: Gastroenterol Clin North Am 1988;17(3):587.

	ABDOMEN
	Peritonitis

Organism	Specimens/Diagnostic Tests	Therapy	Comments
Peritonitis			
Spontaneous or primary (associated with nephrosis or cirrhosis) or peritonitis (SBP): Enterobacteriaceae (GNR) (69%), *S pneumoniae* (GPC), group A *Streptococcus* (GPC), *S aureus* (GPC), anaerobes (5%). Secondary (bowel perforation, hospital-acquired, or antecedent antibiotic therapy): Enterobacteriaceae, *Enterococcus* (GPC), *Bacteroides* sp, *Pseudomonas aeruginosa* (3–15%). Chronic ambulatory peritoneal dialysis: *S epidermidis* (43%), *S aureus* (14%), *Streptococcus* sp (12%), Enterobacteriaceae (14%), *Candida* (2%).	Peritoneal fluid sent for PMN count (86% > 500/μL, 98% specific for SBP), WBC (> 1000/μL, mostly PMNs), pH (< 7.35 in 57%, 96% specific for SBP), Gram's stain (22–77% for SBP) and bacterial culture (65–85% for SBP). (See Ascitic fluid profiles, p 224.) Inoculation of 10 mL of peritoneal fluid into blood culture bottles significantly increases the percentage of positive cultures but is not advised for the Bactec system. Blood cultures for bacteria (aerobic and anaerobic) positive in 75% of SBP cases. Catheter-related infection is associated with a WBC > 500/μL.	Spontaneous or Primary (associated with nephrosis/cirrhosis) (SBP): AMP + APAG or cefoxitin.* Secondary: Cefoxitin or AMP + APAG + Metr.* Associated with chronic ambulatory peritoneal dialysis: Tobramycin (8 mg/L dialysate) + Vanc (25 mg/L dialysate) or TMP/SMX IV or ceftazidime IV.* Ampho + flucytosine if *Candida* sp. Increase the number of exchanges during the first 24 hours to 5 or 6. In many instances, removal of catheter may be avoided.*	In nephrotic patients, Enterobacteriaceae and *S aureus* are most frequent. In cirrhotics, 60% of cases are due to Enterobacteriaceae. "Bacterascites," a positive ascitic fluid culture without an elevated PMN count, is seen in 8% of cases of SBP and probably represents early infection. Ref: Arch Intern Med 1987; 147:73. Ref: Medicine 1987;66:447.

*Adapted and reproduced, with permission, from Sanford JP: *Guide to Antimicrobial Therapy 1991*, Antimicrobial Therapy, Inc, 1991.

ABDOMEN		
Tuberculous Peritonitis/Enterocolitis		
Tuberculous Peritonitis/ Enterocolitis *Mycobacterium tuberculosis* (MTb, AFB, acid-fast beaded rods).	Ascitic fluid for appearance (clear, hemorrhagic or chylous), RBCs (can be high), WBCs (> 1000/µL, > 70% lymphs), protein (> 2.5 g/dL), serum/ascites albumin ratio (< 1.1), AFB stain (rarely positive), culture (< 50% positive). (See Ascitic fluid profiles, p 224.) Culture or AFB smear from other sources (especially from respiratory tract) can help confirm diagnosis. Diagnosis of enterocolitis rests on biopsy of colonic lesions via endoscopy if pulmonary or other extrapulmonary infection cannot be documented. Diagnosis of peritonitis relies upon biopsy of peritoneal lesions via laparoscopy or laparotomy (88%). Operative procedure may be needed to relieve obstruction or for diagnosis.	6-month protocol: INH, Rif, PZA, EMB for 2 months; INH, Rif for remaining 4 months (if sensitivities show MTb sensitive to INH and Rif).	Infection of the intestines can occur anywhere along the GI tract but occurs most commonly in the ileocecal area or mesenteric lymph nodes. It often complicates pulmonary infection. Peritoneal infection usually is an extension of intestinal disease. Symptoms may be minimal even with extensive disease. In the US, 29% of patients with abdominal tuberculosis have a normal chest x-ray. Presence of AFB in the feces does not correlate with intestinal involvement. Ref: Dis Colon Rectum 1987;30:724.

Organism	Specimens/Diagnostic Tests	Therapy	Comments
ABDOMEN			
Diverticulitis			
Enterobacteriaceae (GNR), *Bacteroides* sp, *Enterococcus* (GPC in chains).	Identification of organism is not usually sought. Flat and upright x-rays of abdomen are crucial to rule out perforation (free air under diaphragm) and to localize abscess (air-fluid collections). Barium enema can show presence of diverticuli. Avoid enemas in acute disease because increased intraluminal pressure may cause perforation. Urinalysis will reveal urinary tract involvement, if present.	Principal therapy is an outpatient oral regimen. TMP/SMX + Metr or cefoxitin or Clinda + APAG or Cipr + Metr.*	Pain usually is localized to the left lower quadrant because the sigmoid and descending colon are the most common sites for diverticula. It is important to rule out other abdominal disease (eg, colon carcinoma, Crohn's disease, ischemic colitis). Ref: N Engl J Med 1980; 302:324.
Liver Abscess			
Usually polymicrobial: Enterobacteriaceae (GNR), *Enterococcus* (GPC in chains), *Bacteroides* sp, *S aureus* (GPC in clusters), *Candida* sp, *Entamoeba histolytica*.	CT scan with contrast is the most accurate test to diagnose liver abscess. Antibodies against *E histolytica* should be obtained on all patients. (See Amebic serology, p. 46.) Abscess material obtained via surgery or percutaneous aspiration is recommended for culture when amebic serologies are negative. Chest x-ray is often useful with raised hemidiaphragm, right pleural effusion, or right basilar atelectasis in 41% of patients.	AMP + APAG + Metr or Metr + ceftriaxone.* Open or percutaneous drainage has been very successful in patients with a single bacterial abscess. Amebic abscess: Metr. Drainage is not needed unless abscess is very large or at risk for rupture.*	60% of patients have a single lesion; 40% have multiple lesions. Biliary tract disease is the most common underlying disease, followed by malignancy (biliary tract or pancreatic), colonic disease (diverticulitis), diabetes mellitus, liver disease, and alcoholism. Ref: Medicine 1984;63:291.

*Adapted and reproduced, with permission, from Sanford JP: *Guide to Antimicrobial Therapy 1991*, Antimicrobial Therapy, Inc, 1991.

ABDOMEN		
Cholangitis/Cholecystitis		
Cholangitis/Cholecystitis Enterobacteriaceae (GNR) (68%), *Enterococcus* (GPC in chains) (14%), *Bacteroides* (10%), *Clostridium* sp (GPC) (7%).	Ultrasonography is the best test to quickly demonstrate gallstones or phlegmon around the gallbladder. (See Abdominal ultrasound, p 201.) Radionuclide scans (eg, HIDA, DISIDA) can demonstrate cystic duct obstruction. (See HIDA scan, p 208.) Blood cultures for bacteria (aerobic and anaerobic).	Mezlocillin + Metr or cefoxitin + (APAG or Aztr) or Ceph 3 + (metronidazole or Clinda). Avoid ceftriaxone, which causes biliary concretions.* 15–30% will require decompression (surgical, percutaneous, or endoscopic).* Bowel rest, nasogastric suction, and IV fluids are also mainstays of therapy.*	90% of cases of acute cholecystitis are calculous, 10% are acalculous. Risk factors for acalculous disease include prolonged illness, fasting, hyperalimentation, and carcinoma of the gallbladder or bile ducts. Common bile duct obstruction secondary to tumor or pancreatitis seldom results in infection (0–15%). Ref: Arch Intern Med 1989; 149:1279.

*Adapted and reproduced, with permission, from Sanford JP: *Guide to Antimicrobial Therapy 1991*, Antimicrobial Therapy, Inc, 1991.

	GENITOURINARY		
	Urinary Tract Infection		
Organism	**Specimens/Diagnostic Tests**	**Therapy**	**Comments**
Urinary Tract Infection/Cystitis/Pyuria-Dysuria Syndrome Enterobacteriaceae (GNR, especially *E coli*), *Chlamydia trachomatis, Staphylococcus saprophyticus* (GPC) (in young women), *Enterococcus* (GPC), *N gonorrhoeae* (GNCB), herpes simplex.	Urinalysis and culture reveal the 2 most important signs: bacteriuria ($>10^5$ CFU/mL urine) and pyuria (>10 WBCs/μL). 30% of patients have hematuria. It is generally accepted that $>10^5$ CFU/mL urine represents infection, although women with dysuria and $>10^2$ CFU/mL are also considered to have infection. Intravenous pyelogram and cystoscopy should be performed in women with recurrent or childhood infections, all young boys with UTI, men with recurrent or complicated infection, and patients with symptoms suggestive of obstruction or renal stones. (See Intravenous pyelogram, p 212.)	TMP/SMX or amoxicillin or TMP or doxycycline. Recurrent (>3 episodes/yr): Eradicate infection, then TMP/SMX as long-term or as repeated self-administered single-dose treatment. Single-dose regimens effective in women but have higher early recurrence rates. 3-day regimens have a lower relapse rate and similar side effects as single-dose. A 7-day course is recommended in pregnant women (but TMP/SMX is contraindicated within 2 weeks of due date). Single-dose regimens are inadequate in men. Men with recurrent infections require at least 6 weeks of therapy.	Most men with urinary tract infections have a functional or anatomic genitourinary abnormality. In catheter-related UTI, cure is unlikely unless the catheter is removed. In asymptomatic catheter-related UTI, antibiotics should be given only if patients are at risk for sepsis (old age, underlying disease, diabetes mellitus, pregnancy). Ref: Med Clin North Am 1991; 75(2):313. Ref: Ann Intern Med 1989; 110: 138. Ref: Ann Intern Med 1990; 112: 387.

GENITOURINARY			
		Prostatitis	Pyelonephritis
Prostatitis Acute and Chronic: Enterobacteriaceae (GNR), *Pseudomonas* sp (GNR), *Enterococcus* (GPC in chains).	Urinalysis shows pyuria. Urine culture and Gram's stain usually identify causative organism. Prostatic massage is useful in chronic prostatitis to retrieve organisms but is contraindicated in acute prostatitis (it may cause bacteremia). Bacteriuria is first cleared by treatment with nitrofurantoin or penicillin G. Then urine cultures are obtained from first-void, bladder, and post-prostatic massage urine specimens. A higher organism count in the post-prostatic massage specimen localizes infection to the prostate.	Acute: Cipr or norfloxacin or TMP/SMX or doxycycline or AMP for 14 days. Chronic: FQ for 4–6 weeks results in cure in 80%. TMP/SMX (80 mg/400 mg or "single strength") for 3 months results in improvement in 75%, cure in 33%. Alpha-blocking agents may improve symptoms.	Acute prostatitis is a severe illness characterized by fever, dysuria, and a boggy or tender prostate. Chronic prostatitis often has no symptoms of dysuria or perineal discomfort and a normal prostate exam. Nonbacterial prostatitis (prostatodynia) represents 90% of prostatitis cases. Its etiology is unknown and it is refractory to therapy. Ref: Urology 1990; 36(Suppl 5):13. Ref: Med Clin North Am 1991; 75(2):405.
Pyelonephritis Acute, uncomplicated (usually young women): Enterobacteriaceae (especially *E coli*) (GNR). Complicated (older women, men; post-catheterization, obstruction, post-renal transplant): Enterobacteriaceae (especially *E coli*), *Pseudomonas aeruginosa* (GNR), *Enterococcus* (GPC), *Staphylococcus saprophyticus* (GPC).	Urine culture is indicated when pyelonephritis is suspected. Urinalysis will usually show pyuria and may show WBC casts. Blood cultures for bacteria (aerobic and anaerobic) if sepsis is suspected. Intravenous pyelogram in patients with recurrent infection will show irregularly outlined renal pelvis with caliectasis and cortical scars. (See Intravenous pyelogram, p 212.)	Not septic: PO: TMP/SMX, FQ, Ceph 1.* Septic or Complicated: IV AMP + AG or IV Ceph 1 or APPen or Ceph 3. IV until afebrile for 24–48 hours.* Patients who have no previous episodes of UTI and are mildly ill can be managed as outpatients. In general, patients with nausea and vomiting require hospitalization.*	Patients usually present with fever, chills, nausea, vomiting, and costovertebral angle tenderness. 20–30% of pregnant women with untreated bacteriuria develop pyelonephritis. 25% of *E coli* are resistant to ampicillin in some areas. Ref: Ann Intern Med 1989; 106:341. Ref: Ann Emerg Med 1991; 20: 253.

*Adapted and reproduced, with permission, from Sanford JP: *Guide to Antimicrobial Therapy 1991*, Antimicrobial Therapy, Inc., 1991.

		GENITOURINARY		
Organism		**Specimens/Diagnostic Tests**	**Therapy**	**Comments**

Perinephric Abscess

Organism	Specimens/Diagnostic Tests	Therapy	Comments
Perinephric Abscess Associated with staphylococcal bacteremia: *Staphylococcus aureus* (GPC). Associated with pyelonephritis: Enterobacteriaceae (GNR).	Urinalysis may be normal or may show pyuria. Urine culture (positive in 60%). Blood cultures for bacteria (aerobic and anaerobic) (positive in 20–40%). Bacterial culture of abscess fluid via drainage (percutaneous or surgical). CT scan with contrast is more sensitive than ultrasound in imaging abscess and confirming diagnosis. (See Abdominal CT, p 202.)	Staph bacteremia: PRPen or Ceph 1. Pyelonephritis: IV AMP or IV Ceph 1 or APPen or Ceph 3. IV therapy is given until the patient is afebrile for 24–48 hours. Drainage of the abscess and sometimes partial or complete nephrectomy are required.	Most perinephric abscesses are the result of extension of an ascending urinary tract infection. Often they are very difficult to diagnose. They should be considered in patients who fail to respond to antibiotic therapy, in patients with anatomic abnormalities of the urinary tract, and in patients with diabetes mellitus. Ref: Infect Dis Clin North Am 1987;1(4):907. Ref: Med Clin North Am 1988; 72(5):993.
Urethritis (Gonococcal and Nongonococcal) Gonococcal (GC): *Neisseria gonorrhoeae* (GNDC). Non-gonococcal (NGU): *Chlamydia trachomatis* (50%), *Ureaplasma urealyticum*, *Trichomonas*, herpes simplex, unknown (35%).	Urethral discharge collected with urethral swab shows > 5 WBCs per oil immersion field, Gram's stain (identify gonococcal organisms as gram-negative intracellular diplococci), PMNs (in GC, > 95% of WBCs are PMNs; in NGU usually < 80% are PMNs). Urethral discharge for culture of GC (using Thayer-Martin medium) and *Chlamydia* (cell culture). Urethral discharge can also be tested for chlamydial antigens. VDRL should be checked in all patients because of high incidence of associated syphilis.	GC: Ceftriaxone + doxycycline or Tcn. If penicillinase-producing *N gonorrhoeae* are not prevalent, consider AMP + doxycycline. NGU: Doxycycline or Eryth (especially in pregnancy).	About 50% of patients with GC will have concomitant NGU infection. Always treat sexual partners. Recurrence may be secondary to failure to treat partners. Persistent or recurrent episodes with adequate treatment of patient and partners may warrant further evaluation for other causes (eg, prostatitis). Ref: Med Clin North Am 1990;74(6):1543.

GENITOURINARY			
Epididymitis/Orchitis			
Age < 35 years, homosexual men: *Chlamydia trachomatis*, *N gonorrhoeae* (GNDC). Age > 35 years, boys: Enterobacteriaceae (especially *E coli*) (GNR), *Pseudomonas* sp (GNR).	Urinalysis may reveal pyuria. Patients aged > 35 years will often have midstream pyuria and scrotal edema. Culture urine and expressible urethral discharge when present. Prostatic secretions for Gram's stain and bacterial culture are helpful in older patients. When testicular torsion is considered, Doppler ultrasound or radionuclide scan can be useful in diagnosis.	Age < 35 years: Ceftriaxone + doxycycline or spectinomycin + doxycycline or Cipr + doxycycline. Age > 35 years: TMP/SMX or sulfonamides or AMP or doxycycline. Bed rest and scrotal elevation are recommended until fever and local inflammation have subsided. Failure to improve in 3 days mandates reevaluation and possible hospitalization.	Testicular torsion is a surgical emergency that is often confused with orchitis or epididymitis. Sexual partners should be examined for signs of sexually transmitted diseases. In non-sexually transmitted disease, evaluation for underlying urinary tract infection or structural defect is recommended. Ref: Med Clin North Am 1990;74(6):1543.
Vaginitis/Vaginosis			
Candida sp, *Trichomonas vaginalis*, *Gardnerella vaginalis*, *Bacteroides* (non-*fragilis*), *Mobiluncus*, *Peptostreptococcus* (GPC).	Vaginal discharge for appearance (in candidiasis, area is pruritic with thick "cheesy" discharge; in trichomoniasis, copious foamy discharge), pH (about 4.5 for *Candida*; 5.0–6.0 with bacterial; 5.0–7.0 in *Trichomonas*; KOH preparation (hyphae in *Candida*; "fishy" odor on reaction with *Gardnerella* infection), saline ("wet") preparation (motile organisms seen in *Trichomonas*; cells covered with organisms — "clue" cells—in *Gardnerella*). (See Vaginitis table, p. 245.) Atrophic vaginitis is seen in postmenopausal patients, often with bleeding, scant discharge, and pH 6.0–7.0. Cultures for *Gardnerella* are not useful and are not recommended.	*Candida* sp: Miconazole or clotrimazole or nystatin intravaginally. Avoid intercourse for 1–2 weeks. *Trichomonas vaginalis*: PO Metr. Contraindicated in first trimester of pregnancy (use 20% saline douche instead). Treat male partners. Atrophic: Estrogen cream. Bacterial: PO Metr or Clinda. Treatment of male sexual partners is not needed.	Bacterial vaginosis results from massive overgrowth of vaginal bacterial flora. The etiology is unknown. Serious infectious sequelae associated with bacterial vaginosis include abscesses, endometritis, and pelvic inflammatory disease. There is also a danger of premature rupture of the membranes and premature labor. Ref: Med Clin North Am 1990;74(6):1573. Ref: Rev Infect Dis 1990;12 (Suppl 6):S665.

Organism	Specimens/Diagnostic Tests	Therapy	Comments
GENITOURINARY			
Cervicitis			
Cervicitis, Mucopurulent *Chlamydia trachomatis* (50%), *N gonorrhoeae* (GNDC) (8%).	Cervical swab specimen for appearance (yellow or green purulent material), Gram's stain (for identification of GC), cell count (> 10 WBCs per high-power oil immersion field seen in 91% of *C trachomatis*), and culture (for GC). If GC culture is negative, treat for *C trachomatis*.	GC: Ceftriaxone + Tcn or spectinomycin + doxycycline or Cipr + doxycycline. *C trachomatis*: Tcn or Eryth. Male sexual partners should be treated.	Mucopurulent discharge may persist for 3 months or more even after appropriate therapy. Ref: Sex Transmit Dis 1989;16:103. Ref: Am J Obstet Gynecol 1987; 157:65.
Salpingitis			
Salpingitis/Pelvic Inflammatory Disease (PID) Usually polymicrobial: *N gonorrhoeae* (GNDC), *Chlamydia trachomatis*, *Bacteroides*, *Peptostreptococcus* and other anaerobes, Enterobacteriaceae (GNR), streptococci (GPC in chains), *Mycoplasma hominis* (debatable).	Gram's stain of urethral or endocervical exudate can be diagnostic of gonococcal infection and can be confirmed with culture on Thayer-Martin medium. Endometrial biopsy is sensitive and specific for endometritis. Laparoscopy is the most specific test to confirm the diagnosis of PID. VDRL should be checked in all patients because of high incidence of associated syphilis.	Outpatient (Temperature <38°C, WBC < 11,000/μL, minimal or no peritonitis, active bowel sounds, able to tolerate PO intake): Ceftriaxone + doxycycline or cefoxitin + probenecid + (doxycycline or Eryth). Inpatient: Cefoxitin + doxycycline or Clinda + gentamicin. Patients should be hospitalized when diagnosis is uncertain; pelvic abscess is suspected; pregnant; peritonitis is present; or failure to respond to outpatient therapy after 72 hours.	PID typically progresses from cervicitis to endometritis to salpingitis. PID is a sexually transmitted disease in some cases, not in others. All sexual partners should be examined. All IUDs should be removed. Some recommend that all patients with PID be hospitalized. Ref: Am J Obstet Gynecol 1991;164 (5 Part 2):1370. Ref: Med Clin North Am 1990; 74(6):1603. Ref: JAMA 1991; 266:2594.

BONE		
Osteomyelitis		
Osteomyelitis *Staphylococcus aureus* (GPC) (about 60% of all cases). Infant: *S aureus*, Enterobacteriaceae (GNR), groups A and B streptococci (GPC). Child (<3 years): *H influenzae* (GNCB), streptococci. Child (>3 years) to Adult: *S aureus*. Postoperative: *S aureus*, Enterobacteriaceae, *Pseudomonas* sp (GNR). Joint prosthesis: *S epidermidis*.	Blood cultures for bacteria (aerobic and anaerobic) are positive in about 60%. Percutaneous needle biopsy or open bone biopsy is needed if blood cultures are negative and osteomyelitis is suspected. Imaging with bone scan or gallium scan (sensitivity 95%, specificity 60–70%) can localize areas of suspicion. Plain bone films are abnormal in acute cases after about 2 weeks of illness (33%). Myelography or MRI is indicated to rule out epidural abscess in vertebral osteomyelitis.	Bed rest and 4-6 weeks of parenteral antibiotics. Infant: PRPen + Ceph 3. Child (<3 years): Cefuroxime or Ceph 3. Child (>3 years) to Adult: PRPen. Postoperative: Cipr or TC/CL or Vanc + Ceph 3 or IMP. Joint prosthesis: Vanc. Debridement should be considered if poor response after 48 hours, if soft tissue abscess, or if septic arthritis is present.	Hematogenous or contiguous infection (eg, infected prosthetic joint, chronic cutaneous ulcer) may lead to osteomyelitis in children (metaphyses of long bones) or adults (vertebrae, metaphyses of long bones). Hematogenous osteomyelitis in drug addicts occurs in unusual locations (vertebrae, clavicle, ribs). In infants, osteomyelitis is often associated with contiguous joint involvement. Ref: N Engl J Med 1980; 303:360.

	JOINT		
	Bacterial/Septic Arthritis		
	Organism	Specimens/Diagnostic Tests	Therapy	Comments

Organism	Specimens/Diagnostic Tests	Therapy	Comments
Bacterial/Septic Arthritis Infant (< 3 months): *S aureus* (GPC), Enterobacteriaceae (GNR), group B *Streptococcus* (GPC). Child (3 months to 6 years): *S aureus* (35%), *H influenzae* (GNCB) (15%), *Streptococcus* (10%), Enterobacteriaceae (6%). Adult, venereal disease not likely: *S aureus* (40%), group A *Streptococcus* (27%), Enterobacteriaceae (23%). Adult, venereal disease likely: *N gonorrhoeae* (GNCB) (disseminated gonococcal infection, DGI). Prosthetic joint, postoperative or following intraarticular injection: *S epidermidis* (40%), *S aureus* (20%), Enterobacteriaceae, *Pseudomonas* sp.	Joint aspiration (synovial) fluid for WBCs (in nongonococcal infection, mean WBC is 100,000/μL), Gram's stain (best on centrifuged concentrated specimen), culture (nongonococcal infection in adults [85–95%], DGI [25%]). (See Synovial fluid profiles, p 238.) Blood cultures for bacteria (aerobic and anaerobic) may be useful, especially in infants; nongonococcal infection in adults (50%); DGI (1–3%). DGI may be diagnosed by positive culture from a nonarticular source and by a compatible clinical picture. Gram's stain of skin lesions is rarely positive.	Infant (< 3 months): PRPen + Ceph 3 or PRPen + APAG. Child (3 months to 6 years): (PRPen or Ceph 1 or Vanc) + Ceph 3. Adult, venereal disease not likely: (PRPen or Ceph 1) + APAG or TC/CL. Adult, venereal disease likely: Ceph 3 or spectinomycin. Prosthetic joint, postoperative, or following intraarticular injection: Vanc + (APAG or Aztr) or IMP. Drainage of an infected joint is required. Serial needle drainage once or twice daily is often sufficient. Surgical drainage is needed for hip joints. Prosthetic joint infection requires surgical removal of prosthesis.	Septic arthritis is usually hematogenously acquired. Diminished host defenses secondary to cancer, liver disease, hypogammaglobulinemia are common associations. Nongonococcal bacterial arthritis is usually monarticular (and typically affects one knee joint). DGI is the most common cause of septic arthritis in urban centers and is usually polyarticular with associated tenosynovitis. Ref: Medicine 1983;62:395. Ref: N Engl J Med 1985; 312: 764. Ref: Ann Intern Med 1987; 107: 692.

	MUSCLE	SKIN
	Gas Gangrene	**Impetigo**
Gas Gangrene *Clostridium perfringens* (GPR), other *Clostridium* sp.	Diagnosis should be suspected in areas of devitalized tissue when gas is discovered by palpation (subcutaneous crepitation) or x-ray. Gram's stain of foul-smelling, brown/blood-tinged watery exudate can be diagnostic with gram-positive rods and a remarkable absence of neutrophils. Anaerobic culture of discharge is confirmatory.	Surgical debridement is primary therapy. HD IV Pen G or Metr.* Therapy should be started if clinical picture includes sudden onset of pain, edema, and gas around or within a wound.	Gas gangrene occurs in the setting of a contaminated wound. Infections with *Enterobacter* or *E coli* and anaerobic infections can also cause gas formation. These agents cause cellulitis rather than myonecrosis. Ref: Med J Australia 1984; 140:256.
Impetigo Infant (impetigo neonatorum): *Staphylococcus* (GPC). Nonbullous or "vesicular": Group A *Streptococcus* (GPC), *S aureus* (GPC). Bullous: *S aureus*.	Gram's stain and Tzanck smear of scrapings from lesions may be useful in differentiating impetigo from other vesicular or pustular lesions (herpes simplex, varicella-zoster, contact dermatitis). Tzanck preparation can be performed by scraping the contents, base, and roof of vesicle and applying to glass slide. After fixing, the slide is stained with Wright's or Giemsa's stain and inspected for giant cells. (See Tzanck smear, p 30.)	Infant: PRPen or Vanc.* Nonbullous: Pen V or Eryth or Ceph 1.* Bullous: Dicloxacillin or Eryth or PO Ceph 1.* Topical antibiotics (topical mupirocin 2% or bacitracin) is as effective as Eryth or dicloxacillin in primary and secondary skin infections.*	Impetigo neonatorum requires prompt treatment and protection of other infants (isolation). Ref: J Am Acad Dermatol 1986;14:535.

*Adapted and reproduced, with permission, from Sanford JP: *Guide to Antimicrobial Therapy 1991*, Antimicrobial Therapy, Inc, 1991.

| | SKIN | |
| | Cellulitis | |
Organism	**Specimens/Diagnostic Tests**	**Therapy**	**Comments**
Cellulitis	Skin culture: In spontaneous cellulitis, isolation of the causative organism is difficult. In traumatic and postoperative wounds, Gram's stain may allow rapid diagnosis of staphylococcal or clostridial infection. Culture of wound or abscess material will almost always yield the diagnosis.	Spontaneous, traumatic wound (without sepsis): PO Ceph 1 or dicloxacillin.* Traumatic wound (with sepsis): AM/SB or TC/CL or PRPen + APAG + Clinda. Postoperative wound (not GI or GU): IV Ceph 1 + APAG or PRPen + APAG.*	Cellulitis has long been considered to be the result of an antecedent bacterial invasion with subsequent bacterial proliferation. However, the difficulty in isolating putative pathogens from cellulitic skin has cast doubt on this theory.
Spontaneous, traumatic wound: Polymicrobial: *S aureus* (GPC), groups A, C, D anaerobic streptococci (GPC), Enterobacteriaceae (GNR), *Clostridium perfringens* (GPR), *Clostridium tetani*, *Pseudomonas* sp (GNR) (if water exposure).		Postoperative wound (GI or GU): Cefoxitin or Clinda + APAG or IMP.* Diabetes mellitus: Cefoxitin or IMP or PRPen + APAG + Clinda.*	Consider updating antitetanus prophylaxis for all wounds. In the diabetic, and in postoperative and traumatic wounds, consider prompt surgical debridement for necrotizing fasciitis. With abscess formation, surgical drainage is the mainstay of therapy and may be sufficient.
Postoperative wound (not GI or GU): *S aureus*, group A *Streptococcus*, Enterobacteriaceae, *Pseudomonas* sp.		Bullous lesions, sea water contaminated abrasion, after eating raw seafood: Tcn + APAG or chloramphenicol.*	Ref: Arch Dermatol 1991; 127:493.
Postoperative wound (GI or GU): must add *Bacteroides* sp, anaerobes, *Enterococcus* (GPC), groups B or C streptococci.		Vein graft donor site: PRPen.* Decubitus ulcers: Topical antibiotic powders and adhesive absorbent bandage (Gelfoam).*	Ref: Arch Phys Med Rehabil 1985;66:177.
Diabetes mellitus: Polymicrobial: Group A *Streptococcus*, *Enterococcus*, *S aureus*, Enterobacteriaceae, anaerobes.		Decubitus ulcers with sepsis: Cefoxitin + APAG or IMP or TC/CL or AM/SB.*	
Bullous lesions, sea water contaminated abrasion, after raw seafood consumption: *Vibrio vulnificus*.		Where methicillin-resistant *S aureus* is common, substitute Vanc for PRPen.*	
Vein graft donor site: *Streptococcus*.			
Decubitus ulcers: Polymicrobial: *S aureus*, anaerobic streptococci, Enterobacteriaceae, *Pseudomonas* sp, *Bacteroides* sp.			

*Adapted and reproduced, with permission, from Sanford JP: *Guide to Antimicrobial Therapy 1991*, Antimicrobial Therapy, Inc, 1991.

BLOOD			
Bacteremia of Unknown Source			
Bacteremia of Unknown Source Neonate (< 4 days): Group B *Streptococcus* (GPC), *E coli* (GNR), *Klebsiella* (GNR), *Enterobacter* (GNR), *S aureus* (GPC). Neonate (> 5 days): add *H influenzae* (GNCB). Child (nonimmunocompromised): *H influenzae*, *S pneumoniae* (GPDC), *N meningitidis* (GNDC), *S aureus*. Adult (nonimmunocompromised): Enterobacteriaceae (GNR), group A or D streptococci, *S pneumoniae*, *Bacteroides* sp, *S aureus*. Adult (IV drug use): *S aureus*. Adult (catheter-related, "line" sepsis): *S aureus*, *S epidermidis*. Adult (splenectomized): *S pneumoniae*, *H influenzae*, *N meningitidis*. Neutropenia (< 500 PMN): Enterobacteriaceae, *Pseudomonas* sp, *S aureus*, *S epidermidis*, viridans group *Streptococcus*.	Blood cultures are mandatory for all patients with fever and no obvious source of infection. Often they are negative, especially in neonates. 10 mL per aerobic/anaerobic set should be drawn at onset of febrile episode. Culture should never be drawn from an IV or from a femoral site.	Neonatal (< 4 days): AMP + AMP or AMP + cefotaxime.* Neonatal (> 5 days): AMP + (cefotaxime or ceftriaxone) or AMP + APAG.* Child (nonimmunocompromised): Cefotaxime or ceftriaxone or PRPen + cefuroxime.* Adult (nonimmunocompromised): AMP + APAG + Clinda or IMP or TC/CL.* Adult (IV drug use): PRPen + APAG or Vanc + APAG.* Adult (catheter-related, "line" sepsis): Vanc or PRPen.* Adult (splenectomized): Ceph 3 or cefuroxime.* Neutropenia: Vanc + APAG + APPen or Vanc + APAG + Ceph 3 or ceftazidime.*	High-dose corticosteroids are not beneficial. Catheter-related infection in patients with long-term venous access (Broviac, Hickman, etc) may be treated successfully without removal of the line. Switching needles during blood cultures does not decrease contamination rates and increases the risk of needle-stick injuries. Ref: N Engl J Med 1987; 317:581. Ref: Pediatr Infect Dis J 1986; 5:6. Ref: N Engl J Med 1986; 315:552.

* Adapted and reproduced, with permission, from Sanford JP: *Guide to Antimicrobial Therapy 1991*, Antimicrobial Therapy, Inc. 1991.

6 Diagnostic Imaging: Test Selection & Interpretation

Susan D. Wall, MD, & Cheryl L. Futerman, MD

HOW TO USE THIS SECTION

Information in this chapter is arranged in anatomic order, from superior to inferior. In a book this size, it would not be feasible to include all available diagnostic tests in one chapter. Instead, we have attempted to summarize the essential features of those examinations that are most frequently ordered in modern clinical practice and those that may be associated with difficulty or risk. Indications, advantages and disadvantages, contraindications, and patient preparation are presented. Costs of the studies are approximate and represent averages reported from several large medical centers.

Risks of Intravenous Contrast Studies

While intravenous contrast is an important tool in radiology, it is not without substantial risks. Minor reactions (nausea, vomiting, hives) occur in about 5–10% of patients. Major reactions (laryngeal edema, bronchospasm, cardiac arrest) occur in about 1:3000 patients. Patients at increased risk include those with an allergic history (asthma, hay fever, allergy to foods or drugs). A history of reaction to contrast material is associated with an increased risk of a subsequent severe reaction. Prophylactic measures that may be required in such cases include H_1 and H_2 blockers and corticosteroids.

In addition, there is a risk of contrast-induced renal failure, which is usually mild and reversible. Persons at increased risk for potentially *irreversible* renal damage include those with preexisting renal disease (particularly diabetics with high serum creatinine concentrations), multiple myeloma, severe hyperuricemia, and end-stage heart failure.

In summary, intravenous contrast should be viewed in the same way as other medications—ie, risks and benefits must be weighed before an examination using these pharmaceuticals is ordered.

		HEAD	
		CT	MRI
Test		HEAD **Computed tomography (CT)** $750–$975	HEAD **Magnetic resonance imaging (MRI)** $1300–$1500
Indications		Evaluation of acute craniofacial trauma, acute neurologic dysfunction (<72 hours) from suspected intracranial or subarachnoid hemorrhage. Further characterization of intracranial masses identified by MRI (presence or absence of calcium or involvement of the bony calvarium). Evaluation of sinus disease and temporal bone disease.	Evaluation of essentially all intracranial disease except those listed above for CT.
Advantages		Rapid acquisition makes it the modality of choice for trauma. Superb spatial resolution. Superior to MRI in detection of hemorrhage within the first 24–48 hours.	Provides exquisite spatial resolution, multiplanar capability. Can detect flowing blood and cryptic vascular malformations. Can detect demyelinating and dysmyelinating disease. No beam-hardening artifacts such as can be seen with CT. No ionizing radiation.
Disadvantages/Contraindications		Artifacts from bone may interfere with detection of disease at the skull base and in the posterior fossa. Limited to transaxial views. **Contraindications and risks:** Contraindicated in pregnancy because of the potential harm of ionizing radiation to the fetus. Use of intravenous contrast agents is associated with infrequent but substantial risks (see p 191).	Subject to motion artifacts. Inferior to CT in the setting of acute trauma because it is insensitive to acute hemorrhage, incompatible with life support and traction devices, inferior in detection of bony injury and foreign bodies, and requires longer imaging acquisition time. **Contraindications and risks:** Contraindicated in patients with cardiac pacemakers, intracranial metallic foreign bodies, intracranial aneurysm clips, cochlear implants, some artificial heart valves, and life support devices.
Preparation		Normal hydration. Sedation of agitated patients. Recent serum creatinine determination if intravenous contrast is to be used.	Sedation of agitated patients. Screening CT of the orbits if history suggests possible metallic foreign body in the eye.

	BRAIN		NECK
	Radionuclide scan	**Cisternography**	**MRI**
BRAIN **Brain scan** (radionuclide) $350–$750	Establishment of brain death. Evaluation of suspected herpes simplex encephalitis, dementia, seizures. Single photon emission computed tomography (SPECT) imaging can be used to distinguish ischemia from infarct.	Provides functional information. Can be portable.	Limited resolution. Delayed imaging (1–4 hours) often required. **Contraindications and risks:** Caution in pregnancy because of the potential harm of ionizing radiation to the fetus.	Sedation of agitated patients. Premedicate with potassium perchlorate when using TcO_4 in order to block choroid plexus uptake.
BRAIN **Cisterno-graphy** (radionuclide) $550–$700	Evaluation of hydrocephalus (particularly normal pressure), CSF rhinorrhea or otorrhea, and ventricular shunt patency.	Provides functional information. Can help distinguish normal pressure hydrocephalus from senile atrophy. Can detect CSF leaks.	Requires multiple delayed imaging sessions up to 48–72 hours after injection. **Contraindications and risks:** Caution in pregnancy because of the potential harm of ionizing radiation to the fetus.	Sedation of agitated patients. For suspected CSF leak, pack the patient's nose or ears with cotton pledgets prior to administration of dose. Must follow strict sterile precautions for intrathecal injection.
NECK **Magnetic resonance imaging** (MRI) $1300–$1400	Evaluation of the upper aerodigestive tract. Staging of neck masses. Differentiation of lymphadenopathy from blood vessels. Evaluation of suspected abscess.	Superb spatial resolution and better tissue contrast compared with CT. Sagittal and coronal planar imaging possible. No iodinated contrast needed to distinguish lymphadenopathy from blood vessels.	**Contraindications and risks:** Contraindicated in patients with cardiac pacemakers, intraocular metallic foreign bodies, intracranial aneurysm clips, cochlear implants, some artificial heart valves, and life support devices.	Sedation of agitated patients. Screening CT of orbits if history suggests possible metallic foreign body in the eye.

Test	Indications	Advantages	Disadvantages/Contraindications	Preparation
NECK **Computed tomography** (CT) $1000–$1100	Evaluation of the upper aerodigestive tract. Staging of neck masses. Evaluation of suspected abscess.	Rapid. Superb spatial resolution. Can guide percutaneous fine-needle aspiration of possible tumor or abscess.	Adequate enhancement of vascular structures is mandatory for accurate interpretation. **Contraindications and risks:** Contraindicated in pregnancy because of the potential harm of ionizing radiation to the fetus. Use of intravenous contrast agents is associated with infrequent but substantial risks (see p 191).	Normal hydration. Sedation of agitated patients. Recent serum creatinine determination.
THYROID **Ultrasound** (US) $350–$400	Determination as to whether a palpable nodule is a thyroid nodule and whether single or multiple nodules are present. Assessment of response to suppressive therapy. Screening patients with a history of prior radiation to the head and neck. Guide a biopsy.	Noninvasive. No ionizing radiation. Can be portable. Can image in all planes.	Cannot distinguish between benign and malignant lesions unless local invasion is demonstrated. Technique very operator-dependent. **Contraindications and risks:** None.	None.

THYROID				
Thyroid uptake and scan				
THYROID **Thyroid uptake and scan** (radionuclide) $350–$700	Uptake indicated for evaluation of clinical hypothyroidism, hyperthyroidism, thyroiditis, effects of thyroid-stimulating and suppressing medications, and for calculation of therapeutic radiation dosage. Scanning indicated for above as well as evaluation of palpable nodules, mediastinal mass, and screening of patients with history of head and neck irradiation. Total body scanning used for postoperative evaluation of thyroid metastases.	Demonstrates both morphology and functional information. Can identify ectopic thyroid tissue and "cold" nodules that have a greater risk of malignancy. Imaging of total body with one dose (^{131}I).	Substances interfering with test include iodides in vitamins and medicines, antithyroid drugs, steroids, and intravascular contrast agents. Delayed imaging is required with iodides (^{123}I, 6 hours; ^{131}I total body, 72 hours). Test may not visualize thyroid gland in acute thyroiditis. **Contraindications and risks:** Not advised in pregnancy because of the risk of ionizing radiation to the fetus (iodides cross placenta and concentrate in fetal thyroid). Significant radiation exposure occurs in total body scanning with ^{131}I; patients should be instructed about precautionary measures by nuclear medicine personnel.	Administration of dose after a 4- to 6-hour fast aids absorption. Discontinue all interfering substances prior to test, especially thyroid-suppressing medications: T_3 (1 week), T_4 (4–6 weeks), propylthiouracil (2 weeks).

Test	Indications	Advantages	Disadvantages/Contraindications	Preparation
THYROID — Radionuclide therapy				
THYROID **Thyroid therapy** (radio-nuclide) $50–$300	Treatment of hyperthyroidism and some thyroid carcinomas (papillary and follicular types are amenable to treatment, whereas medullary and anaplastic types are not).	Noninvasive alternative to surgery.	Rarely, radiation thyroiditis may occur 1–3 days after therapy. Hypothyroidism occurs commonly as a long-term complication. Higher doses that are required to treat thyroid carcinoma may result in pulmonary fibrosis. **Contraindications and risks:** Contraindicated in pregnancy and lactation. Contraindicated in patients with metastatic disease to the brain, because treatment may result in brain edema and subsequent herniation, and in those < 20 years of age because of possible increased risk of thyroid cancer later in life. Patients receiving high doses for treatment of thyroid carcinoma must be hospitalized until radioactive level is < 30 mCi.	After treatment, patients must isolate all bodily secretions from household members.
PARATHYROID — Radionuclide scan				
PARATHY-ROID **Parathyroid scan** (radio-nuclide) $400–$500	Evaluation of suspected parathyroid adenoma.	Identifies hyperfunctioning tissue, which is useful when planning surgery.	Small adenomas (< 500 mg) may not be detected. **Contraindications and risks:** Caution in pregnancy is advised because of the risk of ionizing radiation to the fetus.	Requires strict patient immobility during scanning.

CHEST				
Chest radiograph			**CT**	

Test	Indications	Advantages	Disadvantages / Contraindications and risks	Preparation
CHEST **Chest radiograph** $135–$150	Evaluation of pleural and parenchymal pulmonary disease, mediastinal disease, cardiogenic and noncardiogenic pulmonary edema, congenital and acquired cardiac disease. Screening for traumatic aortic rupture (though angiogram is the gold standard). Evaluation of possible pneumothorax (expiratory upright film) or free flowing fluid (decubitus views).	Inexpensive. Widely available.	Difficult to distinguish between causes of hilar enlargement (ie, vasculature vs adenopathy). **Contraindications and risks:** Caution in pregnancy because of the potential harm of ionizing radiation to the fetus.	None.
CHEST **Computed tomography (CT)** $750–$1050	Differentiation of mediastinal and hilar lymphadenopathy from vascular structures. Evaluation and staging of primary and metastatic lung neoplasm. Characterization of pulmonary nodules. Differentiation of parenchymal vs pleural process (ie, lung abscess vs empyema). Evaluation of interstitial lung disease (1.5 mm thin sections), aortic dissection, and aneurysm.	Rapid. Superb spatial resolution. Can guide percutaneous fine-needle aspiration of possible tumor or abscess.	Patient cooperation required for appropriate breath-holding. Generally limited to transaxial views. **Contraindications and risks:** Contraindicated in pregnancy because of the potential harm of ionizing radiation to the fetus. Use of intravenous contrast agents is associated with infrequent but substantial risks (see p 191).	Preferably NPO for 2 hours prior to study. Normal hydration. Sedation of agitated patients. Recent serum creatinine determination.

Test	Indications	Advantages	Disadvantages/Contraindications	Preparation
CHEST **Magnetic resonance imaging** (MRI) $1250–$1350	Evaluation of mediastinal masses. Discrimination between hilar vessels and enlarged lymph nodes. Tumor staging (especially when invasion of vessels or pericardium is suspected). Evaluation of aortic dissection, aortic aneurysm, congenital and acquired cardiac disease.	Provides exquisite spatial resolution, multiplanar capability. No beam-hardening artifacts such as can be seen with CT. No ionizing radiation.	Subject to motion artifacts. **Contraindications and risks**: Contraindicated in patients with cardiac pacemakers, intraocular metallic foreign bodies, intracranial aneurysm clips, cochlear implants, some artificial heart valves, and life support devices.	Sedation of agitated patients. Screening CT of the orbits if history suggests possible metallic foreign body in the eye.
LUNG **Ventilation-perfusion scan** (radionuclide) $400–$500 (ventilation) $450–$500 (perfusion)	Evaluation of pulmonary embolism or burn inhalation injury. Preoperative evaluation of patients with chronic obstructive pulmonary disease and of those who are candidates for pneumonectomy.	Noninvasive. Provides functional information in preoperative assessment.	Patients must be able to cooperate for ventilation portion of the examination. There is a high proportion of indeterminate studies in patients with underlying lung disease. A patient who has a low probability scan still has a 10% chance of having a pulmonary embolus. **Contraindications and risks**: Patients with severe pulmonary artery hypertension or significant right-to-left shunts should have fewer particles injected. Caution advised in pregnancy because of risk of ionizing radiation to the fetus.	Current chest radiograph is mandatory for interpretation.

BREAST **Mammogram** $100–$150	Screening for breast cancer in asymptomatic women: (1) baseline between ages 35 and 40 (at age 30 for women with a first-degree relative with premenopausal breast cancer); (2) every 1–2 years between ages 40 and 49; (3) every year after age 50. If prior history of breast cancer, mammogram should be performed yearly. Indicated at any age for symptoms (palpable mass, bloody discharge) or before planned breast surgery.	Newer film screen techniques generate lower radiation doses (0.1–0.2 rad per film, mean glandular dose).	Detection of breast masses is more difficult in patients with dense breasts. Breast compression may cause patient discomfort. **Contraindications and risks:** Radiation from repeated mammograms can theoretically cause breast cancer; however, the benefits of screening mammograms greatly outweigh the risks.	None.
HEART **Myocardial perfusion scan** (thallium scan) $550–$1250	Evaluation of atypical chest pain. Detection of presence, location, and extent of myocardial ischemia.	Highly sensitive for detecting physiologically significant coronary stenosis. Noninvasive.	The patient must be carefully monitored during treadmill or pharmacologic stress—optimally, under the supervision of a cardiologist. False-positive results may be caused by exercise-induced spasm, aortic stenosis, or left bundle branch block; false-negative results may be caused by inadequate exercise, mild or distal disease, or diffuse ischemia. **Contraindications and risks:** Aminophylline (inhibitor of dipyridamole) is a contraindication to the use of dipyridamole. Treadmill or pharmacologic stress carries a risk of arrhythmia, ischemia, infarct, and, rarely, death. Caution in pregnancy because of the risk of ionizing radiation to the fetus.	Patient should be able to exercise on a treadmill. In case of severe peripheral vascular disease, severe pulmonary disease, or musculoskeletal disorder, pharmacologic stress with dipyridamole may be used. Test should be performed in the fasting state. Patient should not exercise between stress and redistribution.

Test	Indications	Advantages	Disadvantages/Contraindications	Preparation
HEART			**HEART**	
			Pyrophosphate scan	Ventriculography
HEART **Myocardial infarct scan** (pyrophosphate scan) $500–$600	Determination of location and extent of acute myocardial infarction.	Pyrophosphate imaging identifies acute myocardial infarction, including perioperative infarcts following cardiac surgery, where CK and ECG findings may be misleading.	Pyrophosphate scan is most sensitive at 48–72 hours after myocardial injury. Sensitivity is lower for nontransmural infarcts. Sensitivity is also affected by location of infarct (highest for anterior wall, lowest for inferior wall). Pyrophosphate scan may be positive in patients with unstable angina, myocardial contusion, pericarditis, myocarditis, or recent cardioversion. Scan may be persistently positive in up to 20% of patients with remote history of infarct. **Contraindications and risks:** Caution in pregnancy because of the risk of ionizing radiation to the fetus.	Sedation of agitated patients.
HEART **Radionuclide ventriculography** (multigated acquisition [MUGA]) $500–$1,200	Evaluation of patients with ischemic heart disease and other cardiomyopathies. Evaluation of response to pharmacologic therapy and effects of cardiotoxic drugs.	Noninvasive. Resting ejection fraction is a reproducible index that can be used to follow course of disease and response to therapy.	Gated data acquisition may be difficult in patients with severe arrhythmias. Limited to resting study in patients who are unable to exercise on a supine bicycle. **Contraindications and risks:** Recent infarct is a contraindication to exercise ventriculography (arrhythmia, ischemia, infarct, and rarely death may occur with exercise). Caution is advised in pregnancy because of the risk of ionizing radiation to the fetus.	May require harvesting, labeling, and reinjecting the patient's red blood cells. Sterile technique required in handling of red cells.

ABDOMEN		
	KUB	**Ultrasound**
	ABDOMEN **Abdominal plain radiograph** (KUB [Kidneys, ureters, bladder] x-ray) $150–$200	ABDOMEN **Ultrasound** (US) $300–$350
	Assessment of bowel gas patterns (eg, to distinguish ileus from obstruction). To rule out pneumoperitoneum, order an upright abdomen and chest radiograph (acute abdominal series). Good screening test for renal calculi (90% are radiopaque), but not for gallstones (only 15% are radiopaque).	Differentiation of cystic vs solid lesions of the liver and kidneys, intra- and extrahepatic biliary ductal dilatation, cholelithiasis, gallbladder wall thickness, pericholecystic fluid, peripancreatic fluid and pseudocyst, primary and metastatic liver carcinoma, hydronephrosis, abdominal aortic aneurysm, ascites.
	Inexpensive. Widely available.	Noninvasive. No ionizing radiation. Can be portable. Imaging in all planes. Can guide percutaneous fine-needle aspiration of tumor or abscess.
	Supine film alone is inadequate to rule out pneumoperitoneum (see indications). Obstipation may obscure lesions. **Contraindications and risks:** Contraindicated in pregnancy because of the risk of ionizing radiation to the fetus.	Technique very operator-dependent. Organs (particularly pancreas and distal aorta) may be obscured by bowel gas. Presence of barium obscures sound waves. **Contraindications and risks:** None.
	None.	NPO for 6 hours.

| | ABDOMEN |
| | CT |

Test	Indications	Advantages	Disadvantages/Contraindications	Preparation
ABDOMEN **Computed tomography** (CT) $850–$1200	Morphologic evaluation of all abdominal and pelvic organs. Differentiation of intraperitoneal vs retroperitoneal disorders. Evaluation of abscess, trauma, mesenteric and retroperitoneal lymphadenopathy, bowel wall thickening, obstructive biliary disease, pancreatitis, site of gastrointestinal obstruction, pancreatic carcinoma, abdominal aortic aneurysm, splenic infarction, retroperitoneal hemorrhage. Staging of renal cell carcinoma, carcinomas of the GI tract, and metastatic liver disease.	Rapid. Superb spatial resolution. Not limited by overlying bowel gas as with ultrasound. Can guide fine-needle aspiration and percutaneous drainage procedures.	Barium or Hypaque, surgical clips, and metallic prostheses can cause artifacts and degrade image quality. **Contraindications and risks:** Contraindicated in pregnancy because of the potential harm of ionizing radiation to the fetus. Use of intravenous contrast agents is associated with infrequent but substantial risks (see p 191).	Preferably NPO for 4–6 hours. Normal hydration. Opacification of GI tract with water-soluble oral contrast (Gastrografin). Sedation of agitated patients. Recent serum creatinine determination.

ABDOMEN				
MRI				
Magnetic resonance imaging (MRI) $1200–$1400	Clarification of CT findings when surgical clip artifacts are present. Differentiation of retroperitoneal lymphadenopathy from blood vessels or the diaphragmatic crus. Preoperative staging of renal cell carcinoma. Differentiation of benign nonhyperfunctioning adrenal adenoma from malignant adrenal mass. Complementary to CT in evaluation of liver lesions (especially metastatic disease and possible tumor invasion of hepatic or portal veins). Differentiation of benign cavernous hemangioma (> 2 cm in diameter) from malignancy.	Provides exquisite spatial resolution, multiplanar capability. No beam-hardening artifacts such as can be seen with CT. No ionizing radiation.	Subject to motion artifacts. Gastrointestinal opacification not yet readily available. **Contraindications and risks:** Contraindicated in patients with cardiac pacemakers, intraocular metallic foreign bodies, intracranial aneurysm clips, cochlear implants, some artificial heart valves or life support devices.	NPO for 4–6 hours. Intramuscular glucagon to inhibit peristalsis. Sedation of agitated patients. Screening CT of the orbits if history suggests possible metallic foreign body in the eye.

Test	Indications	Advantages	Disadvantages/Contraindications	Preparation
GASTROINTESTINAL				
UGI				
GI **Upper GI study** (UGI) $300–$425	Double-contrast barium technique demonstrates esophageal, gastric, and duodenal mucosa for evaluation of inflammatory disease and other subtle mucosal abnormalities. Single-contrast technique is suitable for evaluation of possible outlet obstruction, peristalsis, gastroesophageal reflux and hiatal hernia, esophageal cancer and varices. Water-soluble contrast (Gastrografin) is suitable for evaluation of anastomotic leak or gastrointestinal perforation.	Good evaluation of mucosa with double-contrast examination. No sedation required. Less expensive than endoscopy.	Aspiration of water-soluble contrast material may occur, inciting severe pulmonary edema. Leakage of barium from a perforation may cause granulomatous inflammatory reaction. Identification of a lesion does not prove it to be the site of blood loss in patients with GI bleeding. Barium precludes endoscopy and body CT examination. Retained gastric secretions prevent mucosal coating with barium. **Contraindications and risks:** Contraindicated in pregnancy because of the potential harm of ionizing radiation to the fetus.	NPO for 8 hours.
GI **Enteroclysis** $500–$575	Barium fluoroscopic study for location of site of intermittent partial small bowel obstruction. Evaluation of extent of Crohn's disease or small bowel disease in patient with persistent gastrointestinal bleeding and normal upper gastrointestinal and colonic evaluations. Evaluation of metastatic disease to the small bowel.	Clarifies lesions noted on more traditional barium examination of the small bowel. Best means of establishing small bowel as normal. Controlled high rate of flow of barium can dilate a partial obstruction.	Requires nasogastric or orogastric tube placement and manipulation to beyond the ligament of Treitz. **Contraindications and risks:** Radiation exposure is substantial, since lengthy fluoroscopic examination is required. Therefore, the test is contraindicated in pregnant women and should be used sparingly in children and women of childbearing age.	Clear liquid diet for 24 hours. Colonic cleansing.

GASTROINTESTINAL	
Peroral pneumocolon	**Barium enema**
GI **Peroral pneumocolon** $50 added to cost of UGI	GI **Barium enema** (BE) $350–$475
Fluoroscopic evaluation of the terminal ileum by insufflating air per rectum after orally ingested barium has reached the cecum.	Double-contrast technique for evaluation of colonic mucosa in patients with suspected inflammatory bowel disease or neoplasm. Single-contrast technique for investigation of possible fistulous tracts, bowel obstruction, large palpable masses in the abdomen, and diverticulitis and for examination of debilitated patients.
Best evaluation of the terminal ileum. Can be performed concurrently with upper GI series.	Good mucosal evaluation. No sedation required.
Undigested food in the small bowel interferes with the evaluation. **Contraindications and risks:** Contraindicated in pregnancy because of the potential harm of ionizing radiation to the fetus.	Retained fecal material limits study. Requires patient cooperation. Marked diverticulosis precludes evaluation of possible neoplasm in that area. Evaluation of right colon occasionally incomplete or limited by reflux of barium across ileocecal valve and overlapping opacified small bowel. Use of barium delays subsequent colonoscopy and body CT. **Contraindications and risks:** Contraindicated in patients with toxic megacolon and immediately after full-thickness colonoscopic biopsy.
Clear liquid diet for 24 hours.	Colon cleansing with enemas, cathartic, and clear liquid diet (1 day in young patients, 2 days in older patients). Intravenous glucagon (which inhibits peristalsis) is given to distinguish colonic spasm from a mass lesion.

Test	Indications	Advantages	Disadvantages/Contraindications	Preparation
GASTROINTESTINAL				
GI **Hypaque enema** $350–$375	Water-soluble contrast for fluoroscopic evaluation of sigmoid or cecal volvulus, anastomotic leak or other perforation. Differentiation of colonic versus small bowel obstruction. Therapy for obstipation.	Water-soluble contrast medium is evacuated much faster than barium because it does not adhere to the mucosa. Therefore, Hypaque enema can be followed immediately by oral ingestion of barium for evaluation of possible distal small bowel obstruction.	Demonstrates only colonic morphologic features and not mucosal changes. Contraindications and risks: Contraindicated in patients with toxic megacolon. Hypertonic solution may lead to fluid imbalance in debilitated patients and children.	Colonic cleansing is desirable but not always necessary.
GI **Esophageal reflux study** (radionuclide) $450–$600	Evaluation of heartburn, regurgitation, recurrent aspiration pneumonia.	Noninvasive and well tolerated. More sensitive for reflux than fluoroscopy, endoscopy, and manometry; similar sensitivity to acid reflux test. Permits quantitation of reflux. Can also identify aspiration into the lung fields.	Incomplete emptying of esophagus may mimic reflux. Abdominal binder—used to increase pressure in the lower esophagus—may not be tolerated in patients who have undergone recent abdominal surgery. Contraindications and risks: Contraindicated in pregnancy because of the potential harm of ionizing radiation to the fetus.	NPO for 4-6 hours. During test, patient must be able to consume 300 mL of liquid.

GASTROINTESTINAL				
Gastric emptying study				**GI bleeding scan**
GI **Gastric emptying study** (radionuclide) $375–$550	Evaluation of dumping syndrome, vagotomy, gastric outlet obstruction due to inflammatory or neoplastic disease, effects of drugs, and other causes of gastroparesis (eg, diabetes mellitus).	Gives functional information not available by other means.	Reporting of meaningful data requires adherence to standard protocol and establishment of normal values. **Contraindications and risks:** Contraindicated in pregnancy because of the potential harm of ionizing radiation to the fetus.	NPO for 4–6 hours. During test, patient must be able to eat a 300-g meal consisting of both liquids and solids.
GI **GI bleeding scan** (labeled red cell or sulfur colloid scan, radionuclide) $600–$800	Evaluation of upper or lower GI blood loss.	Noninvasive compared to angiography. Longer period of imaging possible, which aids in detection of intermittent bleeding. Both labeled red cells and sulfur colloid can detect bleeding rates as low as 0.05–0.10 mL/min (angiography requires rate of about 0.5 mL/min). Labeled red cell scan is more sensitive but less specific than sulfur colloid for detecting GI bleeding.	Bleeding must be active during time of imaging. **Sulfur colloid:** Imaging time limited to approximately 1 hour, whereas red cells can be imaged for up to 24 hours. Upper GI bleeding can be obscured by liver and spleen activity. **Labeled red cells:** Longer imaging time required because of higher background activity. Presence of free TcO_4 (poor labeling efficiency) can lead to gastric, kidney, and bladder activity that can be misinterpreted as sites of bleeding. **Contraindications and risks:** Contraindicated in pregnancy because of the potential harm of ionizing radiation to the fetus.	Sterile technique required during in vitro labeling of red cells.

		GALLBLADDER	
		Ultrasound	**HIDA scan**
Test		GALL-BLADDER **Ultrasound (US)** $200	GALL-BLADDER **99mTc N-substituted iminodiacetic acid (dimethyl-iminodiacetic acid [HIDA] scan)** $450–$550
Indications		Demonstrates cholelithiasis (95% sensitive), gallbladder wall thickening, pericholecystic fluid, intra- and extrahepatic biliary dilatation.	Evaluation of suspected acute cholecystitis or common bile duct obstruction. Evaluation of bile leaks, biliary atresia, and biliary enteric bypass patency.
Advantages		Noninvasive. No ionizing radiation. Can be portable. Imaging in all planes. Can guide fine-needle aspiration, percutaneous transhepatic cholangiography, and biliary drainage procedures.	Hepatobiliary function assessed. Rapid. Not dependent on intestinal absorption. Can be performed in patients with elevated serum bilirubin. No intravenous contrast used.
Disadvantages/Contraindications		Technique very operator-dependent. Presence of barium obscures sound waves. Difficult in obese patients. **Contraindications and risks:** None.	Does not demonstrate the cause of obstruction (eg, tumor or gallstone). Not able to evaluate biliary excretion if hepatocellular function is severely impaired. May require up to 24 hours to distinguish acute from chronic cholecystitis. Sensitivity may be lower in acalculous cholecystitis. False-positive results can occur with hyperalimentation, prolonged fasting, and acute pancreatitis. **Contraindications and risks:** Contraindicated in pregnancy because of the potential harm of ionizing radiation to the fetus.
Preparation		Preferably NPO for 6 hours to enhance visualization of gallbladder.	NPO for 4–6 hours. Some radiologists premedicate patients with cholecystokinin.

	GALLBLADDER Oral cholecystogram			PANCREAS/BILIARY TREE ERCP

Test / Cost	Indications	Advantages	Disadvantages	Preparation
GALLBLADDER **Oral cholecystogram** (OCG) $250	Fluoroscopic evaluation of suspected cholelithiasis when clinical symptoms are highly suggestive but the ultrasound is normal or equivocal. Can assess gallbladder function and possible chronic cholecystitis.	Wide availability. Complements ultrasound.	Test sensitivity depends on intestinal absorption and liver function. Nonvisualization of the gallbladder can be caused by other factors besides obstruction of the cystic duct (eg, Telepaque tablets not absorbed by the gut). Requires up to 24–48 hours to perform. Nausea, vomiting, diarrhea, or headache occurs in up to 50% of patients. Exposure to ionizing radiation. **Contraindications and risks:** Contraindicated in pregnancy because of the potential harm of ionizing radiation to the fetus. Cannot be performed in patients with elevated bilirubin (> 3 mg/dL).	Iopanoic acid (Telepaque) or tyropanoate sodium (Bilopaque) is taken orally the night before the exam. Test may be repeated in 24 hours for "double-dose" examination if gallbladder is not visualized initially.
PANCREAS/BILIARY TREE **Endoscopic retrograde cholangiopancreatography** (ERCP) $600–$650	Primary sclerosing cholangitis, AIDS-associated cholangitis, and cholangiocarcinomas. Demonstrates cause, location, and extent of extrahepatic biliary obstruction (eg, choledocholithiasis). Can diagnose chronic pancreatitis.	Avoids surgery. If stone is suspected, ERCP offers therapeutic potential (sphincterotomy and extraction of common bile duct stone). Finds gallstones in up to 14% of patients with symptoms but negative ultrasound and oral cholecystogram.	Requires endoscopy. May cause pancreatitis (1%), cholangitis (< 1%), peritonitis, hemorrhage (if sphincterotomy performed), and death (rare). **Contraindications and risks:** Contraindicated in patients with concurrent or recent (< 6 weeks) acute pancreatitis. Relatively contraindicated in pancreatic pseudocyst. Contraindicated in pregnancy because of the potential harm of ionizing radiation to the fetus.	NPO for 6 hours. Sedation usually required.

Test	Indications	Advantages	Disadvantages/Contraindications	Preparation
LIVER **Ultrasound** (US) $200	Differentiation of cystic vs solid intrahepatic lesions. Evaluation of intra- and extrahepatic biliary dilatation, primary and metastatic liver tumors, and ascites.	Noninvasive. No radiation. Can be portable. Imaging in all planes. Can guide fine-needle aspiration, percutaneous transhepatic cholangiography, and biliary drainage procedures.	Technique very operator-dependent. Presence of barium obscures sound waves. More difficult in obese patients. **Contraindications and risks**: None.	Preferably NPO for 6 hours.
LIVER, SPLEEN **Liver, spleen scan** (radionuclide) $550–$750	Evaluation of metastatic or primary tumor, inflammatory process, palpable mass, organomegaly, elevated hepatic enzymes, alcoholic liver disease, and thrombocytopenia. Assist in location of an accessory spleen or suspected subphrenic abscess.	Better sampling and more sensitive than ultrasound. May detect isodense lesions missed by CT. Reproducible means of following response to chemotherapy.	Diminished sensitivity for small lesions (less than 1.5–2 cm) and deep lesions. Single photon emission computed tomography (SPECT) increases sensitivity (can detect lesions of 1–1.5 cm). Nonspecific; unable to distinguish solid vs cystic or inflammatory vs neoplastic tissue. Lower sensitivity for diffuse hepatic tumors. **Contraindications and risks**: Caution in pregnancy advised because of the risk of ionizing radiation to the fetus.	None.

	PANCREAS		ADRENAL
	CT	**Ultrasound**	**MIBG scan**
PANCREAS / **Computed tomography (CT)** / $850–$1200	Evaluation of biliary obstruction and possible adenocarcinoma. Staging of pancreatic carcinoma. Diagnosis and staging of acute pancreatitis.	Best means of imaging the pancreas. Can guide fine-needle biopsy or placement of a drainage catheter. Can identify early necrosis in pancreatitis.	Optimal imaging requires intravenous contrast and thin section imaging (5 mm contiguous cuts). **Contraindications and risks:** Contraindicated in pregnancy because of the potential harm of ionizing radiation to the fetus. Use of intravenous contrast agents is associated with infrequent but substantial risks (see p 191).	Preferably NPO for 4–6 hours. Normal hydration. Opacification of GI tract with Gastrografin. Sedation of agitated patients. Recent serum creatinine determination.
PANCREAS / **Ultrasound (US)** / $200	Identification of peripancreatic fluid collections, pseudocysts, and pancreatic ductal dilatation.	Noninvasive. No radiation. Can be portable. Imaging in all planes. Can guide fine-needle aspiration or placement of drainage catheter.	Pancreas may be obscured by overlying bowel gas. Technique very operator-dependent. Presence of barium obscures sound waves. **Contraindications and risks:** None.	Preferably NPO for 6 hours.
ADRENAL / **MIBG (metaiodobenzylguanidine) (radionuclide)** / $1,000–$1,400	Suspected pheochromocytoma when CT is negative or equivocal.	Test is useful for localization of pheochromocytomas (particularly extraadrenal).	High radiation dose to adrenal gland. High cost and limited availability of MIBG. Delayed imaging (1–3 days) necessitates return of patient. **Contraindications and risks:** Contraindicated in pregnancy because of the risk of ionizing radiation to the fetus. Because of the relatively high dose of ^{131}I, patients should be instructed about precautionary measures by nuclear medicine personnel.	Administration of Lugol's iodine solution (to block thyroid uptake) prior to and following administration of dose.

GENITOURINARY

Test	Indications	Advantages	Disadvantages/Contraindications	Preparation
GENITOURINARY **Intravenous pyelogram (IVP)** $375–$400	Fluoroscopic evaluation of uroepithelial neoplasm, calculus, papillary necrosis, and medullary sponge kidney. Screening for urinary system injury after trauma.	Best method for evaluating collecting system. Can assess both renal morphology and function.	Suboptimal evaluation of the renal parenchyma. Does not adequately evaluate cause of ureteral deviation. **Contraindications and risks:** Caution in pregnancy is advised because of the risk of ionizing radiation to the fetus. Use of intravenous contrast agents is associated with infrequent but substantial risks (see p 191).	Adequate hydration. Colonic cleansing is preferred but not essential. Recent serum creatinine determination.
GENITOURINARY **Ultrasound (US)** $250–$350	Evaluation of renal morphology, hydronephrosis, size of prostate, and residual urine volume. Differentiation of cystic vs solid renal lesions.	Noninvasive. No radiation. Can be portable. Imaging in all planes. Can guide fine-needle aspiration or placement of drainage catheter.	Technique very operator-dependent. More difficult in obese patients. **Contraindications and risks:** None.	Preferably NPO for 6 hours. Full urinary bladder required for pelvic studies.
GENITOURINARY **Magnetic resonance imaging (MRI)** $1200–$1400	Staging of cancers of the uterus, cervix, and prostate. Can provide additional information in difficult CT cases of cancer of the kidney and urinary bladder.	Provides exquisite spatial resolution, multiplanar capability. No beam-hardening artifacts such as can be seen with CT. No ionizing radiation.	Subject to motion artifacts. Gastrointestinal opacification not yet readily available. **Contraindications and risks:** Contraindicated in patients with cardiac pacemakers, intraocular metallic foreign bodies, intracranial aneurysm clips, cochlear implants, some artificial heart valves, and life support devices.	Sedation of agitated patients. Screening CT of the orbits if history suggests possible metallic foreign body in the eye.

	GENITOURINARY Radionuclide scan			PELVIS Ultrasound
GENITOURINARY **Renal scan** (radio-nuclide) $550–$750	Evaluation of renal blood flow and function in acute or chronic renal failure. Evaluation of both medical and surgical complications of renal transplant. Estimation of glomerular filtration rate (GFR) and effective renal plasma flow (ERPF). Determination of relative renal function prior to nephrectomy. Parenchymal agents useful in assessment of obstruction. Captopril used in suspected renovascular hypertension.	Provides functional information without risk of iodinated contrast used in IVP. Provides quantitative information not available by other means.	Finding of poor renal blood flow does not pinpoint an etiologic diagnosis. Limited utility when renal function is extremely poor. Estimation of GFR and ERPF often is inaccurate. One- to 4-hour delayed images are necessary with parenchymal agents. Parenchymal agents are nonspecific and do not give information about solid vs cystic nature of lesions. **Contraindications and risks:** Caution in pregnancy because of the risk of ionizing radiation to the fetus.	Relatively high radiation dose with ^{131}I Hippuran, so that good hydration and frequent bladder emptying are advised.
PELVIS **Ultrasound** (US) $300–$350	Evaluation of palpable ovarian mass, enlarged uterus, vaginal bleeding, pelvic pain, possible ectopic pregnancy, and infertility. Monitoring of follicular development. Localization of intrauterine device.	Use of a vaginal probe enables very early detection of intra-uterine pregnancy and ectopic pregnancy and does not require a full bladder.	Vaginal probe has limited field of view and therefore may miss large masses outside the pelvis. **Contraindications and risks:** None.	Distended bladder required (only in transabdominal examination).

	PELVIS			
	MRI			
Test	Indications	Advantages	Disadvantages/Contraindications	Preparation
PELVIS **Magnetic resonance imaging (MRI)** $1200–$1400	Evaluation of gynecologic malignancies, particularly endometrial, cervical, and vaginal carcinoma. Evaluation of prostate, bladder, and rectal carcinoma. Evaluation of congenital anomalies of the genitourinary tract. Useful in distinguishing lymphadenopathy from vasculature.	Provides exquisite spatial resolution, multiplanar capability. No beam-hardening artifacts such as can be seen with CT. No ionizing radiation.	Subject to motion artifacts. **Contraindications and risks:** Contraindicated in patients with cardiac pacemakers, intraocular metallic foreign bodies, intracranial aneurysm clips, cochlear implants, some artificial heart valves, and life support devices.	Intramuscular glucagon is used to inhibit intestinal peristalsis. Air is used in some cases to distend the rectum. Sedation of agitated patients. Screening CT of orbits if history suggests possible metallic foreign body in the eye.

BONE				
Bone scan				
BONE **Bone scan, whole body** (radionuclide) $600–$775	Evaluation of primary or metastatic neoplasm, osteomyelitis, arthritis, metabolic disorders, trauma, avascular necrosis, joint prosthesis, and reflex sympathetic dystrophy.	Can examine entire osseous skeleton or specific area of interest. Highly sensitive compared with plain film radiography for detection of bone neoplasm. In osteomyelitis, bone scan may be positive much earlier (24 hours) than plain film (10–14 days).	Nonspecific. Correlation with plain film radiographs often necessary. Limited utility in patients with poor renal function. Poor resolution in distal extremities, head, and spine; in these instances, single photon emission computed tomography (SPECT) is often useful. Sometimes difficult to distinguish osteomyelitis from cellulitis or septic joint; dual imaging with gallium or with indium-labeled leukocytes can be helpful. False-negative results for osteomyelitis can occur following antibiotic therapy and within the first 24 hours after trauma. In avascular necrosis, bone scan may be hot, cold, or normal, depending on the stage. **Contraindications and risks:** Caution in pregnancy because of the risk of ionizing radiation to the fetus.	None.

Test	Indications	Advantages	Disadvantages/Contraindications	Preparation
SPINE				
Computed tomography (CT) $700–$1000	Evaluation of structures that are not well visualized on MRI, including ossification of the posterior longitudinal ligament, tumoral calcification, osteophytic spurring, retropulsed bone fragments after trauma. Also used for patients in whom MRI is contraindicated.	Rapid. Superb spatial resolution. Can guide percutaneous fine-needle aspiration of possible tumor or abscess.	Generally limited to transaxial views. MRI unequivocally superior in evaluation of the spine and cord except for conditions mentioned in Indications. Artifacts from metal prostheses degrade images. **Contraindications and risks:** Contraindicated in pregnancy because of the potential harm of ionizing radiation to the fetus. Use of contrast agents for CT myelography is associated with infrequent but substantial risks (see p 191).	Normal hydration. Sedation of agitated patients.
SPINE				
Magnetic resonance imaging (MRI) $1300–$1475	Diseases involving the spine and cord except where CT is superior (ossification of the posterior longitudinal ligament, tumoral calcification, osteophytic spurring, retropulsed bone fragments after trauma).	Provides exquisite spatial resolution, multiplanar capability. No beam-hardening artifacts such as can be seen with CT. No ionizing radiation.	Less useful in detection of calcification, small spinal vascular malformations, acute spinal trauma (because of longer acquisition time, incompatibility with life support devices, and inferior detection of bony injury). Subject to motion artifacts. **Contraindications and risks:** Contraindicated in patients with cardiac pacemakers, intraocular metallic foreign bodies, intracranial aneurysm clips, cochlear implants, some artificial heart valves, and life support devices.	Sedation of agitated patients. Screening CT of orbits if history suggests possible metallic foreign body in the eye.

	MUSCULOSKELETAL MRI			VASCULATURE Ultrasound
MUSCULO-SKELETAL SYSTEM **Magnetic resonance imaging** (MRI) $1200–$1400	Evaluation of joints except where a prosthesis is in place. Extent of primary or malignant tumor (bone and soft tissue). Evaluation of aseptic necrosis, bone and soft tissue infections, marrow space disease, and traumatic derangements.	Provides exquisite spatial resolution, multiplanar capability. No beam-hardening artifacts such as can be seen with CT. No ionizing radiation.	Subject to motion artifacts. Less able than CT to detect calcification, ossification, and periosteal reaction. **Contraindications and risks:** Contraindicated in patients with cardiac pacemakers, intraocular metallic foreign bodies, intracranial aneurysm clips, cochlear implants, some artificial heart valves, and life support devices.	Sedation of agitated patients. Screening CT of the orbits if history suggests possible metallic foreign body in the eye.
VASCULA-TURE **Ultrasound** (US) $250–$400	Evaluation of deep venous thrombosis, patency of extremity grafts, inferior vena cava, portal vein, and hepatic veins. Carotid doppler indicated for symptomatic carotid bruit, atypical transient ischemic attack, monitoring after endarterectomy, and baseline prior to major vascular surgery.	Noninvasive. No radiation. Can be portable. Imaging in all planes.	Technique operator-dependent. Ultrasound not sensitive to detection of ulcerated plaque. May be difficult to diagnose tight stenosis vs occlusion. May be difficult to distinguish acute from chronic deep venous thrombosis. **Contraindications and risks:** None.	None.

	BLOOD
	Indium scan

Test	Indications	Advantages	Disadvantages/Contraindications	Preparation
BLOOD **Leukocyte scan** (indium scan, radionuclide) $700–$875	Evaluation of fever of unknown origin, suspected abscess, pyelonephritis, and osteomyelitis.	Highly specific (98%) for infection (in contrast to gallium). Highly sensitive in detecting abdominal source of infection. In patients with fever of unknown origin, total body imaging is advantageous compared with CT scan or ultrasound. Preliminary imaging as early as 4 hours is possible but less sensitive (30–50% of abscesses are detected at 24 hours).	24-hour delayed imaging may limit its utility in critically ill patients. False-negative scans occur with antibiotic administration or in chronic infection. Perihepatic or splenic infection can be missed because of normal leukocyte accumulation in these organs; liver and spleen scan is necessary adjunct in this situation. False-positive scans occur with swallowed leukocytes, bleeding, indwelling tubes and catheters, surgical skin wound uptake, and bowel activity due to inflammatory processes. Pulmonary uptake is nonspecific and has low predictive value for infection. Patients must be able to hold still during relatively long acquisition times (5–10 minutes). **Contraindications and risks:** Contraindicated in pregnancy because of the hazard of ionizing radiation to the fetus. High radiation dose to spleen.	Leukocytes from the patient are harvested, labeled in vitro, and then reinjected; process requires 1–2 hours. Scanning takes place 24 hours later. Homologous donor leukocytes should be used in neutropenic patients.

7 Diagnostic Tests in Differential Diagnosis

HOW TO USE THIS SECTION

This section shows how diagnostic tests can be helpful in differential diagnosis. Material is presented in tabular form and listed in alphabetical order.

7

Abbreviations used throughout this section include the following:

N = normal

Abn = abnormal

Pos = positive

Neg = negative

↑ = increased or high

↓ = decreased or low

Occ = occasional

Table 7–1. ACID-BASE: Laboratory characteristics of primary single disturbances of acid-base balance.[1]

Disturbance	Acute Primary Change	Arterial pH 7.35–7.45	[K⁺] (meq/L) 3.5–5.0	Anion Gap[2] (meq) 8–12	Clinical Features
Normal	None				None.
Respiratory acidosis	P_{CO_2} retention	↓	↑	N	Dyspnea, polypnea, respiratory outflow obstruction, ↑ anterior-posterior chest diameter, musical rales, wheezes. In severe cases, stupor, disorientation, coma.
Respiratory alkalosis	P_{CO_2} depletion	↑	↓	N or ↓	Anxiety, breathlessness, frequent sighing, lungs usually clear to examination, positive Chvostek and Trousseau signs.
Metabolic acidosis	HCO_3^- depletion	↓	↑ or ↓	N or ↑	Weakness, air hunger, Kussmaul respiration, dry skin and mucous membranes. In severe cases, poor skin turgor, coma, hypotension, death.
Metabolic alkalosis	HCO_3^- retention	↑	↓	N	Weakness, positive Chvostek and Trousseau signs, hyporeflexia.

[1] Reproduced, with permission, from Harvey AM et al (editors): *The Principles and Practice of Medicine*, 22nd ed. Appleton & Lange, 1988.

[2] Anion gap = $[Na^+] - ([HCO_3^-] + [Cl^-]) = 8–12$ meq normally.

Table 7-2. ANEMIA: Diagnosis of common anemias based on red blood cell (RBC) indices.[1]

Type of Anemia	MCV (fL)	MCHC (g/dL)	Common Causes	Common Laboratory Abnormalities	Other Clinical Findings
Microcytic, hypochromic	< 80	< 32	Iron deficiency	Low reticulocyte count, low serum and bone marrow iron, high TIBC.	Mucositis, blood loss.
			Thalassemias	Reticulocytosis, abnormal red cell morphology, normal serum iron levels.	Asian, African, or Mediterranean descent.
			Chronic lead poisoning	Basophilic stippling of RBCs, elevated lead and free erythrocyte protoporphyrin levels.	Peripheral neuropathy, history of exposure to lead.
			Sideroblastic anemia	High serum iron, ringed sideroblasts in bone marrow.	Population of hypochromic RBCs on smear.
Normocytic, normochromic	81–100	32–36	Acute blood loss	Blood in stool.	Recent blood loss.
			Hemolysis	Haptoglobin low or absent, reticulocytosis, hyperbilirubinemia.	Hemoglobinuria, splenomegaly.
			Chronic disease	Low serum iron, TIBC low or low normal.	Depends on cause.
Macrocytic, normochromic	> 101[2]	> 36	Vitamin B_{12} deficiency	Hypersegmented PMNs; low serum vitamin B_{12} levels; achlorhydria.	Peripheral neuropathy, glossitis.
			Folate deficiency	Hypersegmented PMNs; low folate levels.	Alcoholism; malnutrition.
			Liver disease	Mean corpuscular volume usually < 120 fL; normal serum vitamin B_{12} and folate levels.	Signs of liver disease.
			Reticulocytosis	Marked (> 15%) reticulocytosis.	Variable.

[1] Modified, with permission, from Ho MT, Saunders CE (editors): *Current Emergency Diagnosis & Treatment*, 3rd ed. Appleton & Lange, 1990.

[2] If MCV > 120–130, vitamin B_{12} or folate deficiency is likely.

MCV = mean corpuscular volume; **MCHC** = mean corpuscular hemoglobin concentration; **TIBC** = total iron-binding capacity; serum; **PMN** = polymorphonuclear cell.

Table 7–3. ANEMIA, MICROCYTIC: Laboratory evaluation of microcytic, hypochromic anemias.[1]

Diagnosis	MCV (fL)	Serum Iron (µg/dL)	Iron-binding Capacity (µg/dL)	Transferrin Saturation (%)	Serum Ferritin (µg/L)	Free Erythrocyte Protoporphyrin (µg/dL)	Basophilic Stippling	Bone Marrow Iron Stores
Normal	80–100	50–175	250–460	16–60	16–300	< 35	Absent	Present
Iron deficiency anemia	↓	< 30	↑	< 16	< 12	↑	Absent	Absent
Anemia of chronic disease	N or ↓	< 30	N or ↓	N or ↓	N or ↑	↑	Absent	Present
Thalassemia minor	↓	N	N	N	N	N	Usually present	Present

[1] Modified, with permission, from Harvey AM et al (editors): *The Principles and Practice of Medicine,* 22nd ed. Appleton & Lange, 1988.

Table 7–4. ASCITES: Ascitic fluid profiles in various disease states.[1]

Diagnosis	Appearance	Fluid Protein (g/dL)	Fluid Glucose (mg/dL)	WBC and Differential (per μL)	RBC (per μL)	Bacteriologic Gram's Stain & Culture	Cytology	Comments
Normal	Clear	< 3.0	Equal to plasma glucose	< 250	Few or none	Neg	Neg	
TRANSUDATES[2]								
Cirrhosis	Clear	< 3.0	N	< 250, MN	Few	Neg	Neg	Occ turbid, rarely bloody. Fluid LDH/Serum LDH ratio < 0.6.
Congestive heart failure	Clear	< 2.5	N	< 250, MN	Few	Neg	Neg	
Nephrotic syndrome	Clear	< 2.5	N	< 250, MN	Few	Neg	Neg	
Pseudo-myxoma peritonei	Gelatinous	< 2.5	N	< 250	Few	Neg	Occ Pos	
EXUDATES[3]								
Bacterial peritonitis	Cloudy	> 3.0	< 50 with perforation	> 500, PMN	Few	Pos	Neg	Blood cultures frequently positive.
Tuberculous peritonitis	Clear	> 3.0	< 60	> 500, MN	Few, occ many	Stain Pos in 25%; culture Pos in 65%	Neg	Occ chylous. Peritoneal biopsy positive in 65%.

Malignancy	Clear or bloody	> 3.0	< 60	> 500, MN, PMN	Many	Neg	Pos in 60–90%	Occ chylous. Fluid LDH/Serum LDH ratio > 0.6. Peritoneal biopsy diagnostic.
Pancreatitis	Clear or bloody	> 2.5	N	> 500, PMN, MN	Many	Neg	Neg	Occ chylous. Fluid amylase > 1000 IU/L, sometimes > 10,000 IU/L. Fluid amylase > serum amylase.
Chylous ascites	Turbid	Varies, often > 2.5	N	Few	Few	Neg	Neg	Fluid TG > 400 mg/dL (turbid). Fluid TG > serum TG.

[1] Modified, with permission, from Harvey AM et al (editors): *The Principles and Practice of Medicine*, 22nd ed. Appleton & Lange, 1988; and Schiff L, Schiff ER (editors): *Diseases of the Liver*, 6th ed. Lippincott, 1987.

[2] Transudates have fluid protein concentration below 2.5–3.0 g/dL; fluid LDH/serum LDH ratio < 0.6 (may be useful in difficult cases).

[3] Exudates have fluid protein concentration above 2.5–3.0 g/dL; fluid LDH/serum LDH ratio > 0.6 (may be useful in difficult cases).

MN = mononuclear cells (lymphocytes or monocytes); **PMN** = polymorphonuclear cells; **CEA** = carcinoembryonic antigen;
TG = triglycerides.

Table 7-5. AUTOANTIBODIES: Associations with connective tissue diseases. [1]

Suspected Disease State	Test	Primary Disease Association (Sensitivity, Specificity)	Other Disease Associations	Comments
CREST syndrome	Anti-centromere antibody	CREST (70–90%, high)	Scleroderma (10–15%), Raynaud's disease (10–30%).	Predictive value of a positive test is > 95% for scleroderma or related disease (CREST, Raynaud's). Diagnosis of CREST is made clinically.
Systemic lupus erythematosus (SLE)	Anti-nuclear antibody (ANA)	SLE (> 95%, low)	RA (30–50%), discoid lupus, scleroderma (60%), drug-induced lupus (100%), Sjögren's syndrome (80%), miscellaneous inflammatory disorders.	Often used as a screening test; a negative test virtually excludes SLE; a positive test, while nonspecific, increases posttest probability. Titer does not correlate with disease activity.
	Anti-double-stranded-DNA (anti-ds-DNA)	SLE (60–70%, high)	Lupus nephritis, rarely RA, CTD, usually in low titer.	Predictive value of a positive test is > 90% for SLE if present in high titer; a decreasing titer may correlate with worsening renal disease. Titer generally correlates with disease activity.
	Anti-Smith antibody (anti-Sm)	SLE (30–40%, high)		SLE-specific. A positive test substantially increases posttest probability of SLE. Test rarely indicated.
Mixed connective tissue disease (MCTD)	Anti-ribonucleo-protein antibody (RNP)	Scleroderma (20–30%, low), MCTD (95–100%, low)	SLE (30%), Sjögren's syndrome, RA (10%), discoid lupus (20–30%).	A negative test essentially excludes MCTD; a positive test in high titer, while nonspecific, increases posttest probability of MCTD.

		Rheumatoid arthritis (RA) (50–90%)	Other rheumatic diseases, chronic infections, some malignancies, some healthy individuals, elderly patients.	Titer does not correlate with disease activity.
Rheumatoid arthritis (RA)	Rheumatoid factor (RF)			
Scleroderma	Anti-Scl-70 antibody	Scleroderma (15–20%, high)		Predictive value of a positive test is > 95% for scleroderma.
Sjögren's syndrome	Anti-SS-A/Ro antibody	Sjögren's (60–70%, low)	SLE (30–40%), RA (10%), subacute cutaneous lupus, vasculitis.	Useful in counseling women of child-bearing age with known CTD, since a positive test is associated with a small but real risk of neonatal SLE and congenital heart block.
Wegener's granulomatosis	Anti-neutrophil cytoplasmic antibody (ANCA)	Wegener's granulomatosis (systemic necrotizing vasculitis) (56–96%, high)	Crescentic glomerulonephritis or other systemic vasculitis (eg, polyarteritis nodosa).	Ability of this assay to reflect disease activity remains unclear.

[1] Modified, with permission, from Harvey AM et al (editors): *The Principles and Practice of Medicine*, 22nd ed. Appleton & Lange, 1988; White RH, Robbins DL: *West J Med* 147, Aug 1987; and Tan EM: *Adv Immunol* 33:173, 1982.
RA = rheumatoid arthritis; **SLE** = systemic lupus erythematosus; **CTD** = connective tissue disease; **MCTD** = mixed connective tissue disease; **SSA** = Sjögren's syndrome A antibody; **CREST** = calcinosis, Raynaud's phenomenon, esophageal dysmotility, sclerodactyly and telangiectasia.

Table 7-6. CEREBROSPINAL FLUID (CSF): CSF profiles in central nervous system disease.[1]

Diagnosis	Appearance	Opening Pressure (mm H$_2$O)	RBC (per μL)	WBC & Diff (per μL)	CSF Glucose (mg/dL)	CSF Protein (mg/dL)	Smears	Culture	Comments
Normal	Clear, colorless	70–200	0	≤ 5MN, 0 PMN	45–85	15–45	Neg	Neg	
Bacterial meningitis	Cloudy	↑↑↑	0	200–20,000, mostly PMN	< 45	> 50	Gram's stain Pos	Pos	PMN predominance may be seen early in course.
Tuberculous meningitis	N or cloudy	↑↑↑	0	100–1000, mostly MN	< 45	> 50	AFB stain Pos	±	
Fungal meningitis	N or cloudy	N or ↑	0	100–1000, mostly MN	< 45	> 50		±	Counterimmunoelectrophoresis or latex agglutination may be diagnostic. CSF and serum cryptococcal antigen positive in cryptococcal meningitis.
Viral (aseptic) meningitis	N	N or ↑	0	100–1000, mostly MN	45–85	N or ↑	Neg	Neg	RBC count may be elevated in herpes simplex encephalitis. Glucose may be decreased in herpes simplex or mumps infections. Viral cultures may be helpful.
Parasitic meningitis	N or cloudy	N or ↑	0	100–1000, mostly MN, E	< 45	N or ↑	Amebae may be seen on wet smear	±	
Carcinomatous meningitis	N or cloudy	N or ↑	0	N or 100–1000, mostly MN	< 45	N or ↑	Cytology Pos	Neg	

Condition	Appearance	Pressure	RBC/µL	Cells/µL	Glucose	Protein	Smear	Culture	Cytology	Comments
Cerebral lupus erythematosus	N	N or ↑	0	N or ↑, mostly MN	N	N or ↑	Neg	Neg	Neg	
Subarachnoid hemorrhage	Pink-red, supernatant yellow	↑	↑ crenated or fresh	N or 100–1000, mostly PMN	N	N op ↑	Neg	Neg	Neg	Blood in all tubes equally. Pleocytosis and low glucose sometimes seen several days after subarachnoid hemorrhage, reflecting chemical meningitis caused by subarachnoid blood.
"Traumatic" tap	Bloody, supernatant clear	N	↑↑↑, fresh	↑	N	↑	Neg	Neg	Neg	Most blood in tube #1, least blood in tube #4.
Spirochetal, early, acute syphilitic meningitis	Clear to turbid	↑	0	25–2000, mostly MN	15–75	> 50	Neg	Neg	Neg	PMN may predominate early. Positive serum RPR or VDRL. CSF VDRL insensitive. If clinical suspicion is high, institute treatment despite negative CSF VDRL.
Late CNS syphilis	Clear	Usually N	0	N or ↑	N	N or ↑	Neg	Neg	Neg	CSF VDRL insensitive (see p 139).
"Neighborhood" meningeal reaction	Clear or turbid, often xanthochromic	Variable, usually N	Variable	↑	N	N or ↑		Usually Neg		May occur in mastoiditis, brain abscess, sinusitis, septic thrombophlebitis, brain tumor, intrathecal drug therapy.
Hepatic encephalopathy	N	N	0	≤ 5	N	N	Neg	Neg	Neg	CSF glutamine > 15 mg/dL.
Uremia	N	Usually ↑	0	N or ↑	N or ↑	N or ↑	Neg	Neg	Neg	
Diabetic coma	N	Low	0	N or ↑	↑	N	Neg	Neg	Neg	

[1] Modified, with permission, from Simon RP et al: *Clinical Neurology*, Appleton & Lange, 1989; Schroeder SA et al: *Current Medical Diagnosis & Treatment 1990*, Appleton & Lange, 1990; and Krupp MA et al: *Physician's Handbook*, Appleton & Lange, 1985. **MN** = mononuclear cells (lymphocytes or monocytes); **PMN** = polymorphonuclear cells; **E** = eosinophils; **CNS** = central nervous system.

Table 7-7. HEMOSTATIC FUNCTION: Laboratory evaluation.[1]

Suspected Diagnosis	Platelet Count	PT	PTT	TT	Further Diagnostic Tests
Idiopathic thrombocytopenic purpura, drug sensitivity, bone marrow depression	↓	N	N	N	Platelet antibody, marrow aspirate.
Disseminated intravascular coagulation	↓	↑	↑	↑	Fibrinogen assays, fibrin D-dimers.
Platelet function defect, salicylates, or uremia	N	N	N	N	Bleeding time, platelet aggregation, blood urea nitrogen (BUN), creatinine.
von Willebrand's disease	N	N	↑ or N	N	Bleeding time, factor VIII assay, factor VIII antigen.
Factor VII deficiency or inhibitor	N	↑	N	N	Factor VII assay (normal plasma should correct PT if no inhibitor is present).
Factor V, X, II, I deficiencies as in liver disease or with anticoagulants	N	↑	↑	N or ↑	Liver function tests.
Factor VIII (hemophilia), IX, XI, or XII deficiencies or inhibitor	N	N	↑	N	Inhibitor screen, individual factor assays.
Factor XIII deficiency	N	N	N	N	Urea stabilizing test, factor XIII assay.

[1] Modified, with permission, from May HL (editor): *Emergency Medicine.* Wiley & Sons, 1984.

Note: In approaching patients with bleeding disorders, try to distinguish clinically between platelet disorders (eg, patient has petechiae, mucosal bleeding) and factor deficiency states (eg, patient has hemarthrosis).

PT = prothrombin time; **PTT** = activated partial thromboplastin time; **TT** = thrombin time.

Table 7–8. HEPATIC FUNCTION TESTS.[1]

Clinical Condition	Direct Bilirubin (mg/dL)	Indirect Bilirubin (mg/dL)	Urine Bilirubin	Serum Albumin & Total Protein (g/dL)	Alkaline Phosphatase (IU)	Prothrombin time (seconds)	ALT (SGPT) AST (SGOT) (IU)
Normal	0.1–0.3	0.2–0.7	None	Albumin, 3.4–4.7. Total protein, 6.0–8.0.	30–115 (lab specific)	11–15 seconds. After vitamin K, 15% increase within 24 hours.	ALT, 5–35 AST, 5–40 (lab-specific)
Hepatocellular jaundice (eg, viral, alcoholic hepatitis)	⇈	↑	↑	↓ Albumin	N to ↑	Prolonged if damage is severe. Does not respond to parenteral vitamin K.	Increased in hepatocellular damage, viral hepatitides; AST/ ALT ratio often > 2:1 in alcoholic hepatitis
Uncomplicated obstructive jaundice (eg, CBD obstruction)	⇈	↑	↑	N	↑	Prolonged if obstruction marked but responds to parenteral vitamin K.	N to minimally ↑
Hemolysis	N	↑	None	N	N	N	N
Gilbert's syndrome	N	↑	None	N	N	N	N
Intrahepatic cholestasis (drug-induced)	⇈	↑	↑	N	⇈	N	AST N or ↑ ALT N or ↑
Primary biliary cirrhosis	⇈	↑	↑	N ↑ globulin	⇈	N or ↑	↑

[1] Modified, with permission, from Schroeder SA et al (editors): *Current Medical Diagnosis & Treatment 1991.* Appleton & Lange, 1991; and Harvey AM et al (editors): *The Principles and Practice of Medicine,* 22nd ed. Appleton & Lange, 1988
AST = aspartate aminotransferase; **ALT** = alanine aminotransferase; **CBD** = common bile duct.

Table 7–9. PLEURAL FLUID: Pleural fluid profiles in various disease states. [1]

Diagnosis	Gross Appear-ance	Protein (g/dL)	Glucose[2] (mg/dL)	WBC and Differential (per μL)	RBC (per μL)	Micro-scopic Exam	Culture	Comments
Normal	Clear	1–1.5	Equal to serum	≤ 1000; mostly MN	0 or Few	Neg	Neg	
TRANSUDATES[3]								
Congestive heart failure	Serous	< 3; sometimes ≥ 3	Equal to serum	< 1000	< 10,000	Neg	Neg	Most common cause of pleural effusion. Effusion right-sided in 55–70% of patients.
Nephrotic syndrome	Serous	< 3	Equal to serum	< 1000	< 1000	Neg	Neg	Occurs in 20% of patients. Cause is low protein osmotic pressure.
Hepatic cirrhosis	Serous	< 3	Equal to serum	< 1000	< 1000	Neg	Neg	From movement of ascites across diaphragm. Treatment of underlying ascites usually sufficient.
EXUDATES[3]								
Tuberculosis	Usually serous; can be bloody	90% ≥ 3; may exceed 5 g/dL	Equal to serum; Occ < 60	500–10,000; mostly MN	< 10,000	Concentrate Pos for AFB in < 50%	May yield MTb	PPD usually positive; pleural biopsy positive; eosinophils (> 10%) or mesothelial cells (> 5%) make diagnosis unlikely.
Malignancy	Usually turbid, bloody; Occ serous	90% ≥ 3	Equal to serum; < 60 in 15% of cases	1000–100,000; mostly MN	> 100,000	Pos cytology in 50%	Neg	Eosinophils uncommon; fluid tends to reaccumulate after removal.

	Appearance		Glucose[2]	WBC count/µL	RBC/µL			Comments
Empyema	Turbid to purulent	≥3	Less than serum, often < 20	25,000–100,000, mostly PMN	< 5,000	Pos	Pos	Drainage necessary; putrid odor suggests anaerobic infection.
Parapneumonic effusion, uncomplicated	Clear to turbid		Equal to serum	5000–25,000, mostly PMN	< 5,000	Neg	Neg	Tube thoracostomy unnecessary; associated infiltrate on chest x-ray; fluid pH ≥ 7.2.
Pulmonary embolism, infarction	Serous to grossly bloody	≥3	Equal to serum	1000–50,000, MN or PMN	100 > 100,000	Neg	Neg	Variable findings; 25% are transudates.
Rheumatoid arthritis or other collagen-vascular disease	Turbid or yellow-green	≥3	Very low (< 40 in most); in RA, 5–20 mg/dL	1000–20,000, mostly MN	< 1000	Neg	Neg	Rapid clotting time; secondary empyema common.
Pancreatitis	Turbid to serosanguineous	≥3	Equal to serum	1000–50,000, mostly PMN	1000–10,000	Neg	Neg	Effusion usually left-sided; high amylase level.
Esophageal rupture	Turbid to purulent; red-brown	≥3	Usually low	< 5000–over 50,000, mostly PMN	< 5000	Pos	Pos	Effusion usually left-sided; high fluid amylase level (salivary); pneumothorax in 25% of cases; pH < 6.0 strongly suggests diagnosis.

[1] Modified, with permission, from *Am Rev Respir Dis* 1968;97:479; Schroeder SA et al (editors): *Current Medical Diagnosis & Treatment 1990.* Appleton & Lange, 1990; and Way LW (editor): *Current Surgical Diagnosis & Treatment,* 9th ed. Appleton & Lange, 1991.

[2] Glucose of pleural fluid in comparison to serum glucose.

[3] Exudative pleural effusions meet at least one of the following criteria: (1) pleural fluid protein/serum protein ratio > 0.5; (2) pleural fluid LDH/serum LDH ratio > 0.6; and (3) pleural fluid LDH > 2/3 upper normal limit for serum LDH. Transudative pleural effusions meet none of these criteria. Transudative effusions also occur in myxedema and sarcoidosis.

MN = mononuclear cells (lymphocytes or monocytes); PMN = polymorphonuclear cells; AFB = acid-fast bacilli; MTb = *Mycobacterium tuberculosis*

Table 7–10. PRENATAL DIAGNOSTIC METHODS: Amniocentesis and chorionic villus sampling.[1]

Method	Procedure	Laboratory Analysis	Waiting Time for Results	Advantages	Disadvantages
Amniocentesis	Between the 12th and 16th weeks, and by the transabdominal approach, 10–30 mL of amniotic fluid is removed for cytologic and biochemical analysis. Preceding ultrasound locates the placenta and identifies twinning and missed abortion.	**1. Amniotic fluid:** • Alpha-fetoprotein • Limited biochemical analysis • Virus isolation studies **2. Amniotic cell culture:** • Chromosomal analysis	3–4 weeks	Over 25 years of experience.	Therapeutic abortion, if indicated, must be done in the second trimester. (RhoGam should be given to Rh-negative mothers to prevent sensitization.) Risks (approximately 1%): • Fetal: puncture or abortion. • Maternal: infection or bleeding.
Chorionic villus sampling	Between the 8th and 12th week, and with constant ultrasound guidance, the trophoblastic cells of the chorionic villi are obtained by transcervical or transabdominal endoscopic needle biopsy or aspiration.	**1. Direct cell analysis:** • Chromosomal studies **2. Cell culture:** • Limited biochemical analysis	1–10 days	Over 5 years of investigational experience. Therapeutic abortion, if indicated, can be done in the first trimester.	Risks (approximately 3%): • Fetal: abortion. • Maternal: bleeding and infection (uncommon).

[1] Modified, with permission, from Schroeder SA et al (editors): *Current Medical Diagnosis & Treatment 1990.* Appleton & Lange, 1990.

Table 7–11. PULMONARY FUNCTION TESTS: Interpretation in obstructive and restrictive pulmonary disease.[1]

Tests	Units	Definition	Obstructive Disease	Restrictive Disease
SPIROMETRY				
Forced vital capacity (FVC)	L	The volume that can be forcefully expelled from the lungs after maximal inspiration.	N or ↓	↓
Forced expiratory volume in one second (FEV₁)	L	The volume expelled in the first second of the FVC maneuver.	↓	N or ↓
FEV₁/FVC	%		↓	N or ↑
Forced expiratory flow from 25% to 75% of the forced vital capacity (FEF 25–75%)	L/sec	The maximal midexpiratory airflow rate.	↓	N or ↓
Peak expiratory flow rate (PEFR)	L/sec	The maximal airflow rate achieved in the FVC maneuver.	↓	N or ↑
Maximum voluntary ventilation (MVV)	L/min	The maximum volume that can be breathed in 1 minute (usually measured for 15 seconds and multiplied by 4).	↓	N or ↓
LUNG VOLUMES				
Slow vital capacity (SVC)	L	The volume that can be slowly exhaled after maximal inspiration.	N or ↓	↓
Total lung capacity (TLC)	L	The volume in the lungs after a maximal inspiration.	N or ↑	↓
Functional residual capacity (FRC)	L	The volume in the lungs at the end of a normal tidal expiration.	↑	N or ↑
Expiratory reserve volume (ERV)	L	The volume representing the difference between functional residual capacity and residual volume.	N or ↓	N or ↓
Residual volume (RV)	L	The volume remaining in the lungs after maximal expiration.	↑	N or ↑
RV/TLC ratio	...		↑	N or ↑

[1] Modified, with permission, from Schroeder SA et al (editors): *Current Medical Diagnosis & Treatment 1990*. Appleton & Lange, 1990. **N** = normal; ↓ = less than predicted; ↑ = greater than predicted. Normal values vary according to subject sex, age, body size, and ethnicity.

Table 7–12. RENAL FAILURE: Renal vs Prerenal Azotemia.[1]

	Renal	Prerenal
BUN (mg/dL)	> 20	> 20
Serum creatinine (mg/dL)	> 1.4	> 1.4
BUN/creatinine ratio	10–20	> 20
Urine [Na^+] (meq/L)	> 40	< 20
FE_{Na^+} [2]	> 1%	< 1%, usually < 0.2%
Renal failure index[3]	> 1	< 1
Urine volume (mL/d)	Variable, often > 400	< 400
Urine osmolality (mosm/kg)	< 350	> 500
Urine specific gravity	1.010–1.016	> 1.040

[1] Modified, with permission, from Cogan MG: *Fluid & Electrolytes: Physiology & Pathophysiology*, Appleton & Lange, 1991; and Schroeder SA etal (editors): *Current Medical Diagnosis & Treatment 1991*. Appleton & Lange, 1991.

[2]
$$FE_{Na^+} = \frac{\text{Urine } Na^+/ \text{Plasma } Na^+}{\text{Urine Creatinine/Plasma Creatinine}} \times 100$$

[3]
$$\text{Renal failure index} = \frac{\text{Urine } Na^+}{\text{Urine Creatinine/Plasma Creatinine}}$$

Table 7–13. RENAL TUBULAR ACIDOSIS (RTA): Laboratory diagnosis of renal tubular acidosis.[1]

Clinical Condition	Renal Defect	GFR	Serum $[HCO_3^-]$ (meq/L)	Serum $[K^+]$ (meq/L)	Minimal Urine pH	Associated Disease States	Treatment
Normal	None	N	24–28	3.5–5	4.8–5.2	None	None
Proximal RTA (type II)	Proximal H^+ secretion	N	15–18	↓	< 5.5	Drugs, Fanconi's syndrome, various genetic disorders, dysproteinemic states, secondary hyperparathyroidism, toxins (heavy metals), tubulointerstitial diseases, nephrotic syndrome, paroxysmal nocturnal hemoglobinuria.	$NaHCO_3$ or $KHCO_3$ (10–15 meq/kg/d), thiazides.
Classic distal RTA (type I)	Distal H^+ secretion	N	20–23	↓	> 5.5	Various genetic disorders, autoimmune diseases, nephrocalcinosis, drugs, toxins, tubulointerstitial diseases, hepatic cirrhosis, empty sella syndrome.	$NaHCO_3$ (1–3 meq/kg/d).
Buffer deficiency distal RTA (type III)	Distal NH_3 delivery	↓	15–18	N	< 5.5	Chronic renal insufficiency, renal osteodystrophy, severe hypophosphatemia.	$NaHCO_3$ (1–3 meq/kg/d).
Generalized distal RTA (type IV)	Distal Na^+ reabsorption, K^+ secretion, and H^+ secretion	↓	24–28	↑	< 5.5	Primary mineralocorticoid deficiency (eg, Addison's disease), hyporeninemic hypoaldosteronism (diabetes mellitus, tubulointerstitial diseases, nephrosclerosis, drugs), salt-wasting mineralocorticoid-resistant hyperkalemia.	Fludrocortisone (0.1–0.5 mg/d), dietary K^+ restriction, furosemide (40–160 mg/d), $NaHCO_3$ (1–3 meq/kg/d).

[1] Modified, with permission, from Cogan MG: *Fluid & Electrolytes: Physiology & Pathophysiology.* Appleton & Lange, 1991.
GFR = glomerular filtration rate.

Table 7-14. SYNOVIAL FLUID: Classification of synovial (joint) fluid.[1]

Type of Joint Fluid	Volume (mL)	Viscosity	Appearance	WBC (per µL)	PMNs	Gram's Stain & Culture	Glucose	Comments
Normal	< 3.5	High	Clear, light yellow	< 200	< 25%	Neg	Equal to serum	
Non-inflammatory (Class I)	Often > 3.5	High	Clear, light yellow	200–2000	< 25%	Neg	Equal to serum	Protein 2–3.5 g/dL. Degenerative joint disease, trauma, avascular necrosis, osteochondritis dissecans; osteochondromatosis, neuropathic arthropathy, subsiding or early inflammation, hypertrophic osteoarthropathy, pigmented villonodular synovitis.
Inflammatory (Class II)	Often > 3.5	Low	Cloudy to opaque, dark yellow	3000–100,000	≥ 50%	Neg	> 25, but lower than serum	Protein > 3 g/dL. Rheumatoid arthritis, acute crystal-induced synovitis (gout, pseudogout), Reiter's syndrome, ankylosing spondylitis, psoriatic arthritis, sarcoidosis, arthritis accompanying ulcerative colitis and Crohn's, rheumatic fever, SLE, scleroderma; tuberculous, viral, or mycotic infections. Crystals diagnostic of gout or pseudogout: gout (urate) crystals show negative birefringence; pseudogout (calcium pyrophosphate) show positive birefringence when red compensator filter is used with polarized light microscopy. Phagocytic inclusions in PMNs suggest rheumatoid arthritis (RA cells). Phagocytosis of leukocytes by macrophages seen in Reiter's syndrome.

| Purulent (Class III) | Often > 3.5 | Low | Cloudy to opaque, dark yellow to green | Usually >40,000, often greater than 100,000 | ≥ 75% | Usually positive | < 25, much lower than serum | Pyogenic bacterial infection (eg, *N gonorrhoeae, S aureus*). Bacteria on culture or Gram's-stained smear. Commonest exception: gonococci seen in only about 25% of cases. WBC count and % PMN lower with infections caused by organisms of low virulence or if antibiotic therapy already started. |
| Hemorrhagic (Class IV) | Often > 3.5 | Variable | Cloudy, pink to red | Usually > 2000 | 30% | Neg | Equal to serum | Trauma with or without fracture, hemophilia or other hemorrhagic diathesis, neuropathic arthropathy, pigmented villonodular synovitis, synovioma, hemangioma and other benign neoplasms. Many RBCs found also. Fat globules strongly suggest intra-articular fracture. |

Table 7-15. SYPHILIS: Laboratory diagnosis of syphilis in untreated patients.[1]

Stage	Onset After Exposure	Persistence	Clinical Findings	Sensitivity of VDRL or RPR[2] (%)	Sensitivity of FTA - ABS[3] (%)	Sensitivity of MHA - TP[4] (%)
Primary	21 days (range 10–90)	2–12 wk	Chancre	72	91	50–60
Secondary	6 wk–6 mo	1–3 mo	Rash, condylomata lata, mucous patches, fever, lymphadenopathy, patchy alopecia	100	100	100
Early latent	< 1 yr	Up to 1 yr	Relapses of secondary syphilis	73	97	98
Late latent	> 1 yr	Lifelong unless tertiary syphilis appears	Clinically silent	73	97	98
Tertiary	1 yr until death	Until death	Dementia, tabes dorsalis, aortitis, aortic aneurysm, gummas	77	99	98

[1] Modified, with permission, from Harvey AM et al (editors): *The Principles and Practice of Medicine,* 22nd ed. Appleton & Lange, 1988.

[2] VDRL is a slide flocculation test for nonspecific (anticardiolipin) antibodies, used for screening, quantitation of titer, and monitoring response to treatment; RPR is an agglutination test for nonspecific antibodies, used primarily for screening.

[3] FTA - ABS is an immunofluorescence test for treponemal antibodies utilizing serum absorbed for nonpathogenic treponemes, used for confirmation of infection, not routine screening.

[4] MHA - TP is a microhemagglutination test similar to the FTA - ABS, but one which can be quantitated and automated.

VDRL = Venereal Disease Research Laboratories test; **RPR** = rapid plasma reagin test; **FTA-ABS** = fluorescent treponemal antibody absorption test; **MHA-TP** = microhemagglutination assay for *T. pallidum.*

Table 7-16. ALPHA-THALASSEMIA SYNDROMES.[1,2]

Syndrome	Alpha Globin Genes	Hematocrit	MCV (fL)
Normal	4	N	N
Silent carrier	3	N	N
Thalassemia minor	2	32–40%	60–75
Hemoglobin H disease	1	22–32%	60–75
Hydrops fetalis	0	Fetal death occurs in utero	

[1] Modified, with permission, from Schroeder SA et al (editors): *Current Medical Diagnosis & Treatment 1991*. Appleton & Lange, 1991.
[2] Alpha thalassemias are due primarily to deletion in the alpha globin gene on chromosome 16.

Table 7-17. BETA-THALASSEMIA SYNDROMES: Findings on hemoglobin electrophoresis.[1,2]

Syndrome	Beta Globin Genes	Hb A[3]	Hb A$_2$ [4]	Hb F[5]
Normal	Homozygous beta	97–99%	1–3%	< 1%
Thalassemia minor	Heterozygous beta^0 [6]	80–95%	4–8%	1–5%
	Heterozygous beta$^+$ [7]	80–95%	4–8%	1–5%
Thalassemia intermedia	Homozygous beta$^+$ (mild)	0–30%	0–10%	6–100%
Thalassemia major	Homozygous beta^0	0	4–10%	90–96%
	Homozygous beta$^+$		4–10%	

[1] Modified, with permission, from Schroeder SA et al (editors): *Current Medical Diagnosis & Treatment 1991*. Appleton & Lange, 1991.
[2] Beta thalassemias are usually caused by point mutations in the beta globin gene on chromosome 11 that result in premature chain terminations or defective RNA transcription, leading to reduced or absent beta globin chain synthesis.
[3] Hb A is composed of 2 alpha chains and 2 beta chains: $\alpha_2\beta_2$.
[4] Hb A$_2$ is composed of 2 alpha chains and 2 delta chains: $\alpha_2\delta_2$.
[5] Hb F is composed of 2 alpha chains and 2 gamma chains: $\alpha_2\gamma_2$.
[6] Beta^0 refers to defects that result in absent globin chain synthesis.
[7] Beta$^+$ refers to defects that cause reduced globin chain synthesis.

Table 7–18. THYROID FUNCTION TESTS.[1]

	Total T₄ (µg/dL)	Free T₄ Index (ng/dL)	Total T₃ (ng/dL)	Sensitive Serum TSH (RIA) (µU/mL)	RAI (¹²³I) Uptake (at 24 hours)	Comments & Treatment
Normal[2]	5.0–12	Varies with method	95–190	0.3–5	10–30%	
Hyperthyroidism	↑	↑	↑	→	↑	In TRH stimulation test, TSH shows no response. Thyroid scan shows increased diffuse activity (Graves' disease) vs "hot" areas (hyperfunctioning nodules). Antithyroglobulin and antimicrosomal antibodies and thyroid-stimulating immunoglobulin elevated in Graves' disease.
Hypothyroidism	→	→	↑	Usually ↑ (primary[3] hypothyroidism); rarely ↓ (secondary[4] hypothyroidism)	N or ↓	TRH stimulation test shows exaggerated response in primary hypothyroidism. In secondary hypothyroidism, TRH test helps to differentiate pituitary from hypothalamic disorders. In pituitary lesions, TSH fails to rise after TRH; in hypothalamic lesions, TSH rises but response is delayed. Antithyroglobulin and antimicrosomal antibodies elevated in Hashimoto's thyroiditis.
Hypothyroidism on replacement						
T₄ replacement	N	N	>	N or →	→	TSH ↓ with 0.1–0.2 mg T₄ qd
T₃ replacement	→	→	>	N or ↓	→	TSH ↓ with 50 µg T₃ qd

Euthyroid following injection of radiographic contrast dye	N	N or ↑	N	N	↓	Effects may persist for 2 weeks or longer.
Pregnancy						Effects may persist for 6–10 weeks postpartum. RAI uptake contraindicated in pregnancy.
Hyperthyroid	↑	↑	↑	↓		
Euthyroid	↑	N	N	↑	N	
Hypothyroid	N or ↓	↓	↑		↑	
Oral contraceptives, estrogens, methadone, heroin	↑	N	↑	N	N	Increased serum thyroid-binding globulin.
Glucocorticoids, androgens, phenytoin, L-asparaginase, salicylates (high dose)	↓	N	N or ↓	N	N	Decreased serum thyroid-binding globulin.
Nephrotic syndrome	↓	N	N or ↓	N	N	Loss of thyroid-binding globulin accounts for serum T_4 decrease.
Iodine deficiency	N	N	N	N	↑	Extremely rare in US.
Iodine ingestion	N	N	N	N	↓	Excess iodine may cause hypothyroidism or hyperthyroidism in susceptible individuals.

[1] Modified, with permission, from Leeper RD: *Current Concepts* 1972; 1:1. Courtesy of the Upjohn Co, Kalamazoo, MI.
[2] Normal values vary with laboratory.
[3] Thyroid (end-organ) failure.
[4] Pituitary or hypothalamic lesions.
V = variable.

Table 7–19. URINE COMPOSITION: Urine composition in common disease states.[1]

Disease	Daily Volume	Specific Gravity	Protein[2] (mg/dL)	Ester-ase	Nitrite	RBC	WBC	Casts	Other Microscopic Findings
Normal	600–2500 mL	1.003–1.030	0–trace (0–30)	Neg	Neg	0 or Occ	0 or Occ	0 or Occ	Hyaline casts
Fever	↓	↑	Trace or 1+ (<30)	Neg	Neg	0	Occ	0 or Occ	Hyaline casts, tubular cells
Congestive heart failure	↓	↑ (varies)	1–2+ (30–100)	Neg	Neg	None or 1+	0	1+	Hyaline and granular casts
Eclampsia	↓	↑	3–4+ (30–2000)	Neg	Neg	None or 1+	0	3–4+	Hyaline casts
Diabetic coma	↑ or ↓	↑	1+ (30)	Neg	Neg	0	0	0 or 1+	Hyaline casts
Acute glomerulonephritis	↓	↑	2–4+ (100–2000)	Pos	Neg	1–4+	1–4+	2–4+	Blood; RBC, cellular, granular, and hyaline casts; renal tubular epithelium
Nephrotic syndrome	N or ↓	N or ↑	4+ (>2000)	Neg	Neg	1–2+	0	4+	Granular, waxy, hyaline, and fatty casts; fatty tubular cells
Chronic renal failure	↑ or ↓	Low; invariable	1–2+ (30–100)	Neg	Neg	Occ or 1+	0	1–3+	Granular, hyaline, fatty, and broad casts
Collagen-vascular disease	N,↑ or ↓	N or ↓	1–4+ (30–2000)	Neg	Neg	1–4+	0 or Occ	1–4+	Blood; cellular, granular, hyaline, waxy, fatty, and broad casts; fatty tubular cells; telescoped sediment
Pyelonephritis	N or ↓	N or ↓	1–2+ (30–100)	Pos	Pos	0 or 1+	4+	0 or 1+	WBC casts and hyaline casts; many pus cells; bacteria
Hypertension	N or ↑	N or ↓	None or 1+ (<30)	Neg	Neg	0 or Occ	0 or Occ	0 or 1+	Hyaline and granular casts

[1] Modified, with permission, from Krupp MA et al (editors): *Physician's Handbook,* 21st ed. Lange, 1985.
[2] Protein concentration in mg/dL is listed in parentheses.

Table 7–20. VAGINAL DISCHARGE: Laboratory evaluation of vaginal discharge.[1]

Diagnosis	pH	Odor With KOH (Positive "Whiff" Test)	Epithelial Cells	WBCs	Organisms	KOH Prep	Gram Stain	Comments
Normal	< 4.5	No	N	Occ	Variable, large rods not adherent to epithelial cells	Neg	Gram-positive rods	
Trichomonas vaginalis vaginitis	> 4.5	Yes	N	↑	Motile, flagellated organisms	Neg	Flagellated organisms	
Bacterial vaginosis (*Gardnerella vaginalis*)	> 4.5	Yes	Clue cells[2]	Occ	Coccobacilli adherent to epithelial cells	Neg	Gram-negative coccobacilli	
Candida albicans vaginitis	< 4.5	No	N	Occ slightly increased	Budding yeast or hyphae	Budding yeast or hyphae	Budding yeast or hyphae	Usually white "cottage cheese" curd
Mucopurulent cervicitis (*N gonorrhoeae*)	Variable, usually > 4.5	No	N	↑	Variable	Neg	Intracellular gram-negative diplococci	

[1] Modified, with permission, from Kelly KG: Tests on vaginal discharge. In: Walker HK et al (editors): *Clinical Methods: The History, Physical and Laboratory Examinations,* 3rd ed. Butterworths, 1990.

[2] Epithelial cells covered with bacteria to the extent that cells borders are obscured.

Table 7–21. VALVULAR HEART DISEASE: Diagnostic evaluation of cardiac valvular disease. [1]

Diagnosis	Chest X-ray	ECG	Echocardiography	Comments
MITRAL STENOSIS (MS) Rheumatic disease	Straight left heart border. Large LA sharply indenting esophagus. Elevation of left main bronchus. Calcification occ seen in MV.	Broad negative phase of diphasic P in V_1. Tall peaked P waves, right axis deviation, or RVH appear if pulmonary hypertension is present.	**M-Mode:** Thickened, immobile MV with anterior and posterior leaflets moving together. Slow early diastolic filling slope. LA enlargement. Normal to small LV. **2D:** Maximum diastolic orifice size reduced. Reduced subvalvular apparatus. Foreshortened, variable thickening of other valves. **Doppler:** Prolonged pressure half-time across MV. Indirect evidence of pulmonary hypertension.	"Critical" MS is usually defined as a valve area < 1.0 cm^2. Balloon valvuloplasty has high initial success rates and higher patency rates than for AS. Open commissurotomy can be effective. Valve replacement is indicated when severe regurgitation is present. Catheterization can confirm echo results.
MITRAL REGURGITATION (MR) Myxomatous degeneration (MV prolapse) Infective endocarditis Subvalvular dysfunction Rheumatic disease	Enlarged LV and LA.	Left axis deviation or frank LVH. P waves broad, tall, or notched, with broad negative phase in V_1.	**M-Mode and 2D:** Thickened MV in rheumatic disease. MV prolapse; flail leaflet or vegetations may be seen. Enlarged LV. **Doppler:** Regurgitant flow mapped into LA. Indirect evidence of pulmonary hypertension.	In nonrheumatic MR, valvuloplasty without valve replacement is increasingly successful. Acute MR (endocarditis, ruptured chordae) requires emergent valve replacement. Catheterization is the best assessment of regurgitation.
AORTIC STENOSIS (AS) Calcific (especially in congenitally bicuspid valve) Rheumatic disease	Concentric LVH. Prominent ascending aorta, small knob. Calcified valve common.	LVH.	**M-Mode:** Dense persistent echoes of the AoV with poor leaflet excursion. LVH with preserved contractile function. **2D:** Poststenotic dilatation of the aorta with restricted opening of the leaflets. Bicuspid AoV in about 30%. **Doppler:** Increased transvalvular flow velocity, yielding calculated gradient.	"Critical" AS is usually defined as a valve area < 0.7 cm^2 or a peak systolic gradient of > 50 mm Hg. Catheterization is definitive diagnostic test. Prognosis without surgery is less than 50% survival at 3 yr when CHF, syncope, or angina occur. Balloon valvuloplasty has a high restenosis rate.

AORTIC REGURGITATION (AR) Bicuspid valves Infective endocarditis Hypertension Rheumatic disease Aortic/aortic root disease	Moderate to severe LV enlargement. Prominent aortic knob.	LVH.	**M-Mode** Diastolic vibrations of the anterior leaflet of the MV and septum. Early closure of the valve when severe. Dilated LV with normal or decreased contractility. **2D:** May show vegetations in endocarditis, bicuspid valve, or root dilatation. **Doppler:** Demonstrates regurgitation. Estimates severity.	Aortography at catheterization can demonstrate AR. Acute incompetence leads to LV failure and requires AoV replacement.
TRICUSPID STENOSIS (TS) Rheumatic disease	Enlarged RA only.	Tall, peaked P waves. Normal axis.	**M-Mode and 2D:** TV thickening. Decreased early diastolic filling slope of the TV. MV also usually abnormal. **Doppler:** Prolonged pressure half-time across TV.	Right heart catheterization is diagnostic. Valvulotomy may lead to success, but TV replacement is usually needed.
TRICUSPID REGURGITATION (TR) RV overload (pulmonary hypertension) Inferior infarction Infective endocarditis	Enlarged RA and RV.	Right axis deviation usual.	**M-Mode and 2D:** Enlarged RV. MV often abnormal and may prolapse. **Doppler:** Regurgitant flow mapped into RA and venae cavae. RV systolic pressure estimated.	RA and jugular pressure tracings show a prominent V wave and rapid Y descent. Replacement of TV is rarely done. Valvuloplasty is often preferred.

[1] Modified, with permission, from Schroeder SA et al (editors): *Current Medical Diagnosis & Treatment 1991.* Appleton & Lange, 1991.
RA = right atrium; **RV** = right ventricle; **LA** = left atrium; **LV** = left ventricle; **AoV** = aortic valve; **MV** = mitral valve; **TV** = tricuspid valve; **LVH** = left ventricular hypertrophy; **RVH** = right ventricular hypertrophy; **CHF** = congestive heart failure.

Table 7-22. WHITE BLOOD CELLS: White blood cell count and differential.[1]

Cells	Range (10³/μL)	Increased in	Decreased in
WBC count (total)	3.4–10.0	Infection, hematologic malignancy.	Decreased production (aplastic anemia, folate or B_{12} deficiency, drugs [eg, ethanol, chloramphenicol]); decreased survival (sepsis, hypersplenism, drugs).
Neutrophils	1.8–6.8	Infection (bacterial or early viral), acute stress, acute and chronic inflammation, tumors, drugs, diabetic ketoacidosis, leukemia (rare).	Aplastic anemia, drug-induced neutropenia (eg, chloramphenicol, phenothiazines, antithyroid drugs, sulfonamide), folate or B_{12} deficiency, Chédiak-Higashi syndrome, malignant lymphoproliferative disease, physiologic (in children up to age 4 years).
Lymphocytes	0.9–2.9	Viral infection (especially infectious mononucleosis, pertussis), thyrotoxicosis, adrenal insufficiency, ALL and CLL, chronic infection, drug and allergic reactions, autoimmune diseases.	Immune deficiency syndromes.
Monocytes	0.1–0.6	Inflammation, infection, malignancy, tuberculosis, myeloproliferative disorders.	Depleted in overwhelming bacterial infection.
Eosinophils	0–0.4	Allergic states, drug sensitivity reactions, skin disorders, tissue invasion by parasites, polyarteritis nodosa, hypersensitivity response to malignancy (eg, Hodgkin's disease), pulmonary infiltrative disease, disseminated eosinophilic hypersensitivity disease.	Acute and chronic inflammation, stress, drugs (corticosteroids).
Basophils	0–0.1	Hypersensitivity reactions, drugs, myeloproliferative disorders (eg, CML), myelofibrosis.	

[1] In the automated differential, 10,000 WBCs are classified on the basis of size and peroxidase staining as neutrophils, monocytes, or eosinophils (peroxidase-positive) and as lymphocytes or large unstained cells (LUC), which are peroxidase-negative. LUCs larger than normal lymphocytes, may be atypical lymphocyte or peroxidase-negative blasts. Basophils are identified using two-angle light scattering, based on their singular resistance to lysis.
The reproducibility of 100-cell manual differentials is notoriously poor. Review of blood smears is useful to visually identify rare abnormal cells, blasts, nucleated RBCs, morphologic abnormalities (eg, hypersegmentation, toxic granulation, sickle cells, target cells, spherocytes, basophilic stippling) and to look for rouleaux (stacking of red cells due to increased globulins) and clumped platelets. WBC differential is unlikely to be abnormal with a normal WBC count or to be changed if the total WBC count is unchanged.

8 Diagnostic Algorithms

HOW TO USE THIS SECTION

This section contains algorithms for difficult diagnostic challenges. Decision trees are laid out in an easy-to-read format with diagnostic tests encircled in oval outlines, diagnoses in italics, and therapies in rectangles (see Figure 8–1).

Algorithms are arranged in alphabetical order according to diagnostic topic. Figures included in this section are as follows:

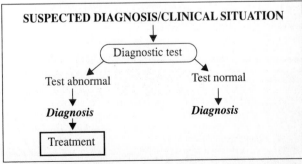

SUSPECTED DIAGNOSIS/CLINICAL SITUATION

Diagnostic test

Test abnormal — *Diagnosis* — Treatment

Test normal — *Diagnosis*

Figure 8–1. ALGORITHM LAYOUT: Diagnostic tests are enclosed in ovals; diagnoses in italics; and treatment recommendations in rectangles.

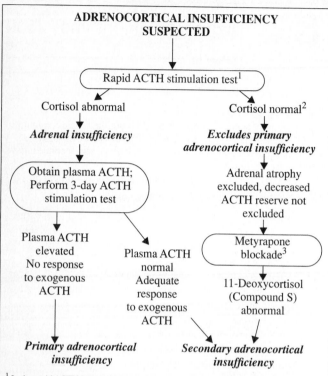

**ADRENOCORTICAL INSUFFICIENCY
SUSPECTED**

Rapid ACTH stimulation test[1]

Cortisol abnormal

Adrenal insufficiency

Obtain plasma ACTH;
Perform 3-day ACTH
stimulation test

Plasma ACTH
elevated
No response
to exogenous
ACTH

Plasma ACTH
normal
Adequate
response
to exogenous
ACTH

*Primary adrenocortical
insufficiency*

Cortisol normal[2]

*Excludes primary
adrenocortical insufficiency*

Adrenal atrophy
excluded, decreased
ACTH reserve not
excluded

Metyrapone
blockade[3]

11-Deoxycortisol
(Compound S)
abnormal

*Secondary adrenocortical
insufficiency*

[1] In the rapid ACTH stimulation test, a baseline cortisol sample is obtained; cosyntropin 0.25 mg is given IM or IV; and plasma cortisol samples are obtained 30 or 60 minutes later.

[2] The normal response is a cortisol increment > 7 μg/dL. If a cortisol level of > 18 μg/dL is obtained, the response is normal regardless of the increment.

[3] Metyrapone blockade is performed by giving 2.0–2.5 g metyrapone PO at 12 midnight. Draw cortisol and 11-deoxycortisol levels at 8 AM. 11-Deoxycortisol level < 7 μg/dL indicates secondary adrenal insufficiency (as long as there is adequate blockade of cortisol synthesis [cortisol level < 10 μg/dL]).

Figure 8–2. ADRENOCORTICAL INSUFFICIENCY: Laboratory evaluation of suspected adrenocortical insufficiency. **ACTH** = adrenocorticotrophic hormone. (Modified, with permission, from Baxter JD, Tyrrell JB: The Adrenal Cortex. In: *Endocrinology and Metabolism.* Felig P et al [editors], McGraw-Hill, 1981; and Harvey AM et al [editors]: *The Principles and Practice of Medicine,* 22nd ed. Appleton & Lange, 1988.)

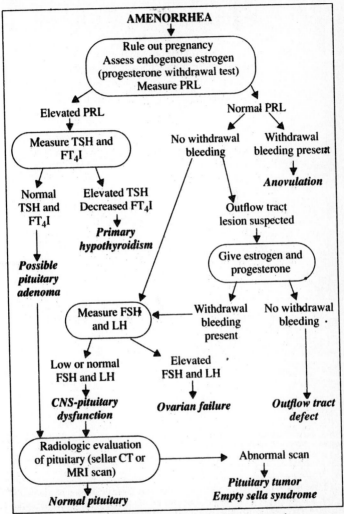

Figure 8–3. AMENORRHEA: Diagnostic evaluation of amenorrhea.
PRL = prolactin; **FT₄I** = free thyroxine index; **TSH** = thyroid stimulating hormone; **FSH** = follicle stimulating hormone; **LH** = luteinizing hormone; **CT** = computed tomography; **MRI** = magnetic resonance imaging. (Modified, with permission, from Greenspan FS [editor]: *Basic and Clinical Endocrinology*, 3rd ed. Appleton & Lange, 1991.)

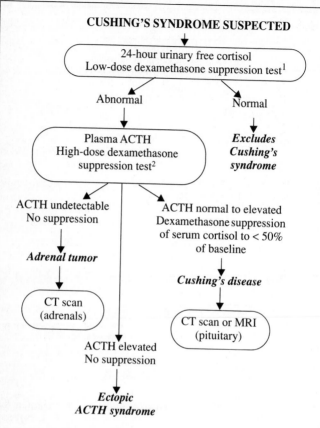

CUSHING'S SYNDROME SUSPECTED

24-hour urinary free cortisol
Low-dose dexamethasone suppression test[1]

Abnormal → Normal

Plasma ACTH
High-dose dexamethasone
suppression test[2]

Normal → *Excludes Cushing's syndrome*

ACTH undetectable
No suppression

Adrenal tumor

CT scan
(adrenals)

ACTH normal to elevated
Dexamethasone suppression
of serum cortisol to < 50%
of baseline

Cushing's disease

CT scan or MRI
(pituitary)

ACTH elevated
No suppression

Ectopic ACTH syndrome

[1] Low dose: Give 1 mg dexamethasone at 11 PM; draw serum cortisol at 8 AM. Normally, AM cortisol is < 5 μg/dL.
[2] High dose: Give 8 mg dexamethasone at 11 PM; draw serum cortisol at 8 AM or collect 24-hour urinary free cortisol. Normally, AM cortisol is < 5 μg/dL.

Figure 8–4. CUSHING'S SYNDROME: Diagnostic evaluation of Cushing's syndrome. **ACTH** = adrenocorticotrophic hormone; **CT** = computed tomography; **MRI** = magnetic resonance imaging. (Modified, with permission, from Baxter JD, Tyrrell JB: The Adrenal Cortex. In: *Endocrinology and Metabolism,* Felig P et al [editors]. 2nd ed. McGraw-Hill, 1987; Harvey AM et al [editors]: *The Principles and Practice of Medicine,* 22nd ed, Appleton & Lange, 1988; and Greenspan FS [editor]: *Basic and Clinical Endocrinology,* 3rd ed. Appleton & Lange, 1991.)

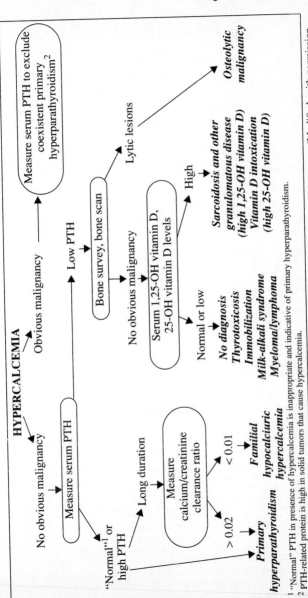

Figure 8-5. HYPERCALCEMIA: Diagnostic approach to hypercalcemia. **PTH** = parathyroid hormone. (Modified, with permission, from Harvey AM et al [editors]: *The Principles and Practice of Medicine,* 22nd ed. Appleton & Lange, 1988.)

1 "Normal" PTH in presence of hypercalcemia is inappropriate and indicative of primary hyperparathyroidism.

2 PTH-related protein is high in solid tumors that cause hypercalcemia.

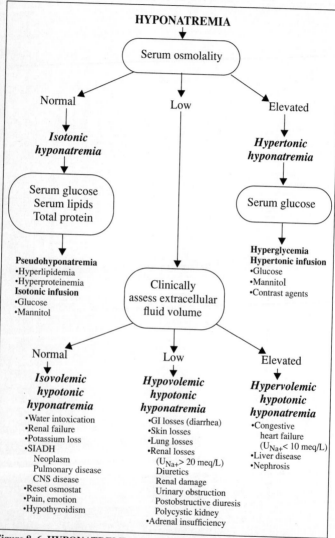

Figure 8–6. HYPONATREMIA: Evaluation of hyponatremia. **SIADH** = syndrome of inappropriate antidiuretic hormone; U_{Na+} = urinary sodium. (Adapted, with permission, from Narins RG et al: *Am J Med* 1982;72:496.)

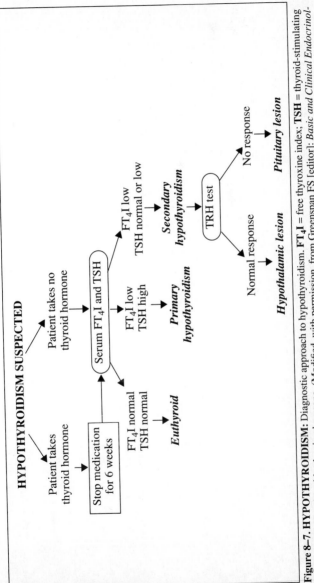

Figure 8–7. HYPOTHYROIDISM: Diagnostic approach to hypothyroidism. **FT₄I** = free thyroxine index; **TSH** = thyroid-stimulating hormone; **TRH** = thyroid-releasing hormone. (Modified, with permission, from Greenspan FS [editor]: *Basic and Clinical Endocrinology*, 3rd ed. Appleton & Lange, 1991.)

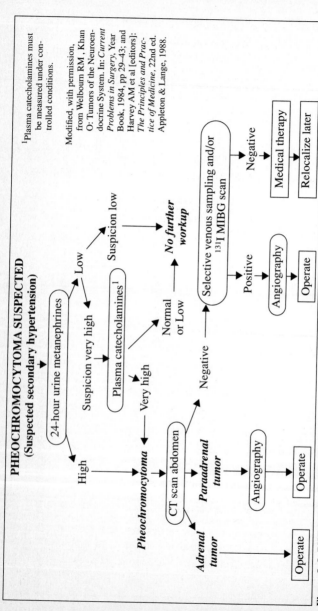

Figure 8–8. PHEOCHROMOCYTOMA: Flow chart for investigation and localization of a possible pheochromocytoma.
^{131}**I MIBG** = ^{131}I metaiodobenzylguanidine.

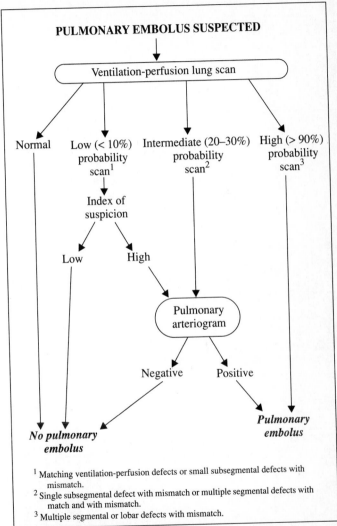

PULMONARY EMBOLUS SUSPECTED

Ventilation-perfusion lung scan

Normal

Low (< 10%) probability scan[1]

Intermediate (20–30%) probability scan[2]

High (> 90%) probability scan[3]

Index of suspicion

Low

High

Pulmonary arteriogram

Negative

Positive

No pulmonary embolus

Pulmonary embolus

[1] Matching ventilation-perfusion defects or small subsegmental defects with mismatch.

[2] Single subsegmental defect with mismatch or multiple segmental defects with match and with mismatch.

[3] Multiple segmental or lobar defects with mismatch.

Figure 8–9. PULMONARY EMBOLUS: Diagnostic evaluation of possible pulmonary embolus. (Modified, with permission, from Wyngaarden JB, Smith LH [editors]: *Cecil's Textbook of Medicine,* 18th ed, Saunders, 1988.)

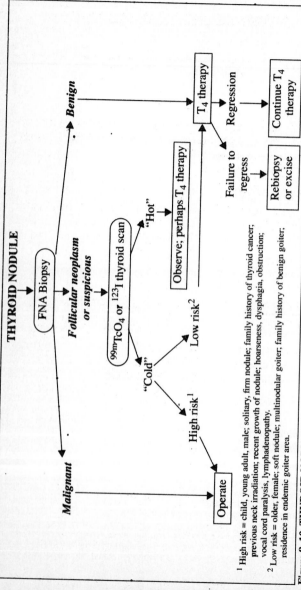

Figure 8–10. THYROID NODULE: Laboratory evaluation of a thyroid nodule. FNA = fine-needle aspiration; T_4 = thyroxine. (Modified, with permission, from Greenspan FS [editor]: *Basic and Clinical Endocrinology* 3rd ed. Appleton & Lange, 1991.)

[1] High risk = child, young adult, male; solitary, firm nodule; family history of thyroid cancer; previous neck irradiation; recent growth of nodule; hoarseness, dysphagia, obstruction; vocal cord paralysis, lymphadenopathy.

[2] Low risk = older, female; soft nodule; multinodular goiter; family history of benign goiter; residence in endemic goiter area.

9 Nomograms & Reference Material

This chapter contains useful laboratory nomograms and reference material. Subjects are presented in alphabetical order and include the following:

Contents **Page**

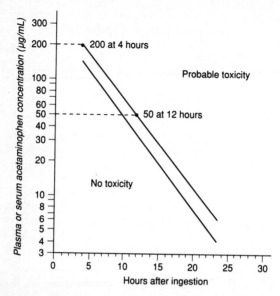

Figure 9–1. ACETAMINOPHEN TOXICITY: Nomogram for prediction of acetaminophen hepatotoxicity following acute overdosage. The upper line defines serum acetaminophen concentrations known to be associated with hepatotoxicity; the lower line defines serum levels 25% below those expected to cause hepatotoxicity. To give a margin for error, the lower line should be used as a guide to treatment. (Modified and reproduced, with permission, from Rumack BM, Matthew M: Pediatrics 1975;55:871; and Ho MT, Saunders CE (editors): *Current Emergency Diagnosis & Treatment*, 3rd ed. Appleton & Lange, 1990.)

Table 9–1. CHILD'S CRITERIA: Relationship of hepatic function and nutrition to operative death rate after portacaval shunt.[1]

	Group		
	A	**B**	**C**
Operative death rate	2%	10%	50%
Serum bilirubin (mg/dL)	< 2	2–3.0	> 3
Serum albumin (g/dL)	> 3.5	3–3.5	< 3
Ascites	None	Easily controlled	Poorly controlled
Encephalopathy	None	Minimal	Advanced
Nutrition	Excellent	Good	Poor

[1] Reproduced, with permission, from Way LW (editor): *Current Surgical Diagnosis & Treatment*, 8th ed. Appleton & Lange, 1988.

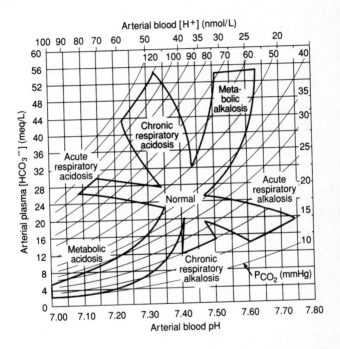

Figure 9–2. ACID-BASE NOMOGRAM: Shown are the 95% confidence limits of the normal respiratory and metabolic compensations for primary acid-base disturbances. (Reproduced, with permission, from Cogan MG (editor): *Fluid and Electrolytes: Physiology and Pathophysiology*. Appleton & Lange, 1991.)

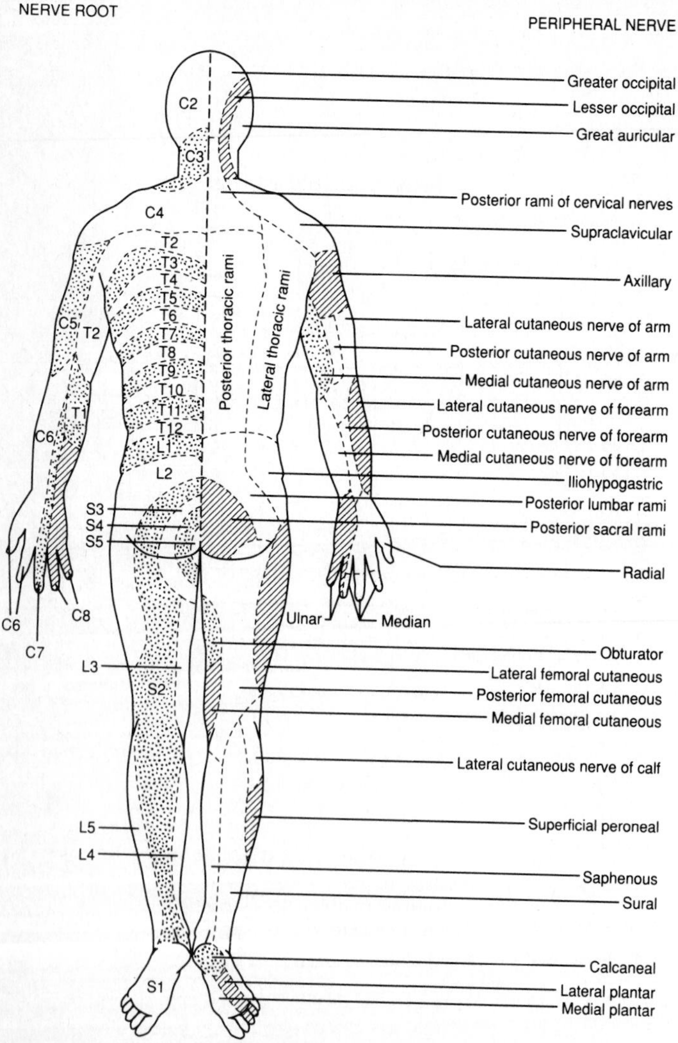

NERVE ROOT

PERIPHERAL NERVE

Figure 9–3. DERMATOME CHART: Cutaneous innervation. The segmental or radicular (root) distribution is shown on the left side of the body and the peripheral nerve distribution on the right side. Above: anterior view; facing page: posterior view. (Reproduced, with permission, from Simon RP et al: *Clinical Neurology.* Appleton & Lange, 1989.)

PERIPHERAL NERVE

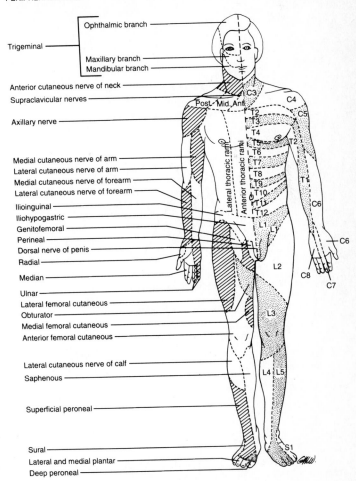

Trigeminal
- Ophthalmic branch
- Maxillary branch
- Mandibular branch

Anterior cutaneous nerve of neck

Supraclavicular nerves

Axillary nerve

Medial cutaneous nerve of arm
Lateral cutaneous nerve of arm
Medial cutaneous nerve of forearm
Lateral cutaneous nerve of forearm

Ilioinguinal
Iliohypogastric
Genitofemoral
Perineal
Dorsal nerve of penis
Radial

Median

Ulnar
Lateral femoral cutaneous
Obturator
Medial femoral cutaneous
Anterior femoral cutaneous

Lateral cutaneous nerve of calf
Saphenous

Superficial peroneal

Sural
Lateral and medial plantar
Deep peroneal

C3 C4 C5
Post. Mid. Ant.
T2 T3 T4 T5 T6 T7 T8 T9 T10 T11 T12
Lateral thoracic rami
Anterior thoracic rami
T2 T1 C6 C6 C8 C7
L1 L1
L2
L3
L4 L5
S1

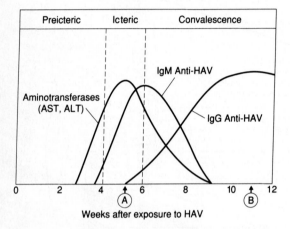

Patterns of Antibody Tests		
	IgM Anti-HAV	IgG Anti-HAV
A Acute HA	+	+ or −
B Convalescence (indicates previous infection)	−	+

Figure 9–4. HEPATITIS A: Usual pattern of serologic changes in hepatitis A. **HA** = hepatitis A; **AST** = aspartate aminotransferase; **ALT** = alanine aminotransferase; **Anti-HAV** = hepatitis A virus antibody; **IgM** = immunoglobulin M; **IgG** = immunoglobulin G. (Reproduced, with permission, from Harvey AM et al (editors): *The Principles and Practice of Medicine*, 22nd ed. Appleton & Lange, 1988.)

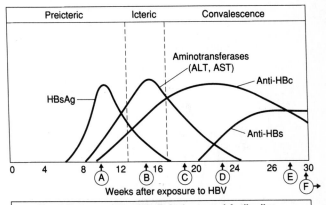

Usual Patterns of Hepatitis B Antigens and Antibodies			
	HBsAg	Anti-HBc	Anti-HBs
A Very Early	+	+ or −	−
B Acute	+	+	−
C Active HB with high titer Anti-HBc ("window")	−	+	−
D Convalescence	−	+	+
E Recovery	−	+ or −	+
F Chronic carrier	+	+	−

Figure 9–5. HEPATITIS B: Usual pattern of serologic changes in hepatitis B. **HBsAg** = hepatitis B surface antigen; **Anti-HBc** = hepatitis B core antibody; **Anti-HBs** = hepatitis B surface antibody; **AST** = aspartate aminotransferase; **ALT** = alanine aminotransferase. (Modified and reproduced, with permission, from Harvey AM et al (editors): *The Principles and Practice of Medicine*, 22nd ed. Appleton & Lange, 1988.)

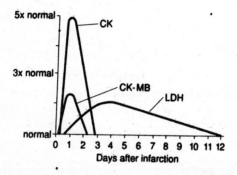

Figure 9–6. MYOCARDIAL ENZYMES: Time course of serum enzyme concentrations after a typical myocardial infarction. **CK** = creatine kinase; **CK-MB** = isoenzyme of CK, which is found mainly in myocardium and is therefore more specific for myocardial damage. **LDH** = lactate dehydrogenase. (Reproduced, with permission, from Harvey AM et al (editors): *The Principles and Practice of Medicine*, 22nd ed. Appleton and Lange, 1988.)

Table 9–2. THE OSMOLAL GAP IN TOXICOLOGY[1]

The osmolal gap (Δ osm) is determined by subtracting the calculated serum osmolality from the measured serum osmolality.

$$\begin{array}{l}\text{Calculated}\\\text{osmolality (osm)}\\(\text{mosm/kg } H_2O)\end{array} = 2\,(Na^+\,[\,meq/L\,]) + \frac{\text{Glucose (mg/dL)}}{18} + \frac{\text{BUN (mg/dL)}}{2.8}$$

Osmolal gap (Δ osm) = Measured osmolality – Calculated osmolality

Serum osmolality may be increased by contributions of circulating alcohols and other low-molecular-weight substances. Since these substances are not included in the calculated osmolality, there will be an osmolal gap directly proportional to their serum concentration and inversely proportional to their molecular weight:

$$\text{Serum concentration (mg/dL)} \approx \Delta\text{ osm} \times \frac{\text{Molecular weight of toxin}}{10}$$

For ethanol (the commonest cause of Δ osm), a gap of 30 mosm/kg H_2O indicates an ethanol level of:

$$30 \times \frac{46}{10} = 138 \text{ mg/dL}$$

See below for lethal concentrations of alcohols and their corresponding osmolal gaps.

Lethal concentrations of alcohols and their corresponding osmolal gaps

	Molecular Weight	Lethal Concentration (mg/dL)	Corresponding Osmolal Gap (mosm/kg H_2O)
Ethanol	46	350	75
Methanol	32	80	25
Ethylene glycol	62	200	35
Isopropanol	60	350	60

Note: Most laboratories use the freezing point method for calculating osmolality. If the vaporization point method is used, alcohols are driven off and their contribution to osmolality is lost.

---

[1] Modified from Ho MT, Saunders CE (editors): *Current Emergency Diagnosis & Treatment*, 3rd ed. Appleton & Lange, 1990.

Na^+ = sodium; **BUN** = blood urea nitrogen.

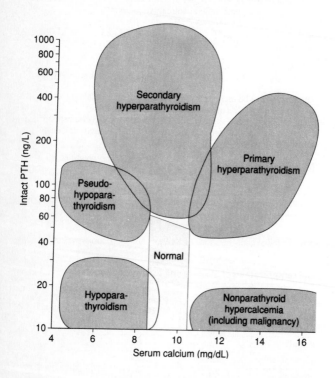

Figure 9–7. PARATHYROID HORMONE & CALCIUM NOMO-GRAM: Relationship between serum intact parathyroid hormone (PTH) and serum calcium levels in patients with hypoparathyroidism, pseudo-hypoparathyroidism, nonparathyroid hypercalcemia, primary hyperpara-thyroidism, and secondary hyperparathyroidism. (Courtesy of GJ Strewler, MD).

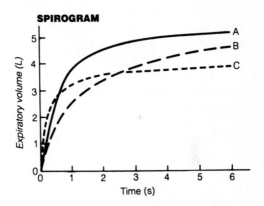

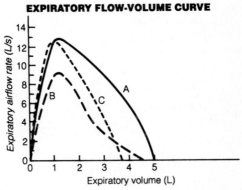

Figure 9–8. PULMONARY FUNCTION TESTS, SPIROMETRY:
Representative spirograms (upper panel) and expiratory flow-volume
curves (lower panel) for normal (**A**), obstructive (**B**), and restrictive (**C**)
patterns. (Reproduced, with permission, from Schroeder SA et al (editors): *Current Medical Diagnosis & Treatment 1990.* Appleton & Lange,
1990.)

Table 9–3. RANSON'S CRITERIA FOR SEVERITY OF ACUTE PANCREATITIS[1]

Criteria present at diagnosis or admission
Age over 55 years
White blood cell count > 16,000/μL
Blood glucose > 200 mg/dL
Serum LDH > 350 IU/L (laboratory-specific)
AST (SGOT) > 250 IU/L (laboratory-specific)

Criteria developing during first 48 hours
Hematocrit fall > 10%
BUN rise > 5 mg/dL
Serum calcium < 8 mg/dL
Arterial PO_2 < 60 mm Hg
Base deficit > 4 meq/L
Estimated fluid sequestration > 6 L

Mortality rates correlate with the number of criteria present:

Number of Criteria	Mortality
0–2	1%
3–4	16%
5–6	40%
7–8	100%

---

[1] Modified from Way LW (editor): *Current Surgical Diagnosis & Treatment*, 8th ed. Appleton & Lange, 1988.
LDH = lactic dehydrogenase; **AST** = aspartate dehydrogenase; **BUN** = blood urea nitrogen.

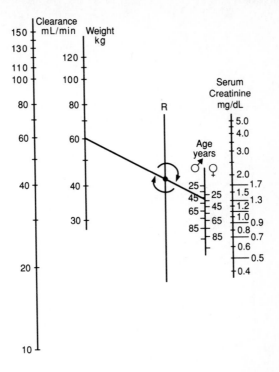

Figure 9–9. RENAL FAILURE: ESTIMATED CREATININE CLEARANCE:
Siersbaek-Nielsen nomogram for estimation of creatinine clearance from serum
creatinine.

• Identify the axis point along the reference line (**R**) around which the relation
between the patient's serum creatinine and creatinine clearance rotates. To do
so, place a straight edge ruler to connect the patient's age (in years, for male or
female) with the patient's weight (in kg).

• Put a dot along the reference line R where the ruler and line intersect.

• Rotate the ruler to connect the patient's serum creatinine and this dot and
determine where the ruler falls along the line estimating the patient's creatinine clearance.

Note: This nomogram is based on the assumption that an increase in weight
represents an increase in lean body mass. Substantial error in the estimate
occurs when a weight increase reflects obesity rather than increased lean body
mass. In addition, the nomogram yields a much more accurate estimate in the
presence of moderate to moderately severe renal impairment than in the presence of normal renal function. It should also not be relied upon in severe renal
insufficiency (eg, serum creatinine > 5 mg/dL or creatinine clearance < 15
mL/min). (Modified, with permission, from Harvey AM et al (editors): The
Principles and Practice of Medicine, 22nd ed. Appleton & Lange, 1988.)

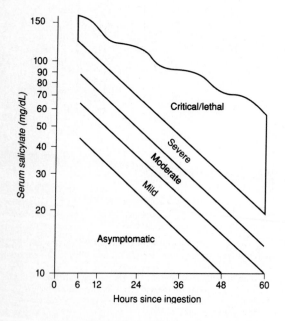

Figure 9–10. SALICYLATE TOXICITY: Nomogram for determining severity of salicylate intoxication. Absorption kinetics assume acute ingestion of non-enteric-coated aspirin preparation. (Modified and reproduced, with permission, from Done AK: Pediatrics 1960;26:800; and Ho MT, Saunders CE (editors): *Current Emergency Diagnosis & Treatment*, 3rd ed. Appleton & Lange, 1990.)

10 Organization of Clinical Data: Pocket Patient Cards

Introduction

One of the constant challenges for health care providers is the collection, synthesis, and dissemination of clinical data. As the practice of medicine becomes increasingly more complicated, physicians and other health care providers are looking for ways to improve their management of patient information. Pocket Patient Cards were designed to help meet this need.

Pocket Patient Cards are 3×5 cards, preprinted with an outline of the standard history and physical (blue card) and a schematic for entry of follow-up laboratory data (orange card). They are designed for medical students, residents, and attending physicians to record details of their ambulatory and hospitalized patients. They are devised to be carried in the shirt pocket so that they can be referred to at any time.

History & Physical Card (Blue)

The front of the history and physical card (Figure 10–1) has room on the top for the patient's addressograph (name, birth date, and hospital identification number), date of admission (DOA), date of discharge (DOD), identifying information (ID), chief complaint (CC), history of present illness (HPI), and problem list. The reverse side (Figure 10–1) has room for past medical history (PMH), family history (FH), social history (SH), physical exam (PE), and standard laboratory data (LAB). This card can be filled out when the patient enters the hospital or the clinic for the first time.

Data Card (Orange)

The front of the data card has room at the top for the patient's name and hospital number as well as space for recording the major test results, problems, and medications used throughout the course of patient care. The remainder of the card is used for daily record keeping—a box for the date, and spaces for temperature (T), blood pressure (BP), pulse (P), respirations (R), weight (Wt), and intake and output (I/O). The remainder of the space is for recording relevant daily laboratory results.

Ordering

Samples of each type of Pocket Patient Card are included with this book. Refills are available in packages of 25 and retail for $2.69. Look for Pocket Patient Cards in your local medical bookstore or write to:

**Pocket Patient
233 Arbor Street
San Francisco, CA 94131**

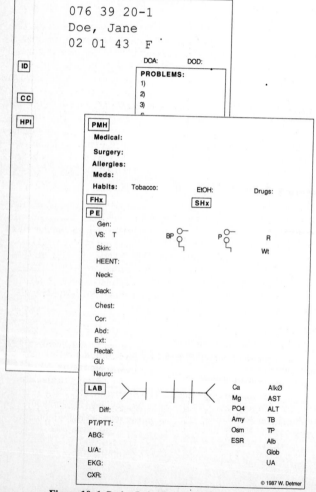

Figure 10–1. Pocket Patient History & Physical Card.

Index

NOTE: Page numbers in boldface type indicate a major discussion. A *t* following a page number indicates tabular material and an *i* following a page number indicates an illustration. Drugs are listed under their generic names.

Notes

Notes

Notes

Notes

Notes

Quick Index